THE ORGAN DONOR PROCESS

THE
ORGAN
DONOR
PROCESS

A Diverse and Global Reward in Recognition of Life Support

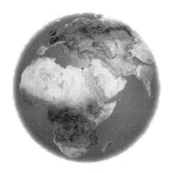

JARED E. EDISON

iUniverse®

THE ORGAN DONOR PROCESS
A DIVERSE AND GLOBAL REWARD IN
RECOGNITION OF LIFE SUPPORT

iUniverse books may be ordered through booksellers or by contacting:

iUniverse
1663 Liberty Drive
Bloomington, IN 47403
www.iuniverse.com
1-800-Authors (1-800-288-4677)

Because of the dynamic nature of the Internet, any web addresses or links contained in this book may have changed since publication and may no longer be valid. The views expressed in this work are solely those of the author and do not necessarily reflect the views of the publisher, and the publisher hereby disclaims any responsibility for them.

Any people depicted in stock imagery provided by Thinkstock are models, and such images are being used for illustrative purposes only.
Certain stock imagery © Thinkstock.

ISBN: 978-1-4917-6710-8 (sc)
ISBN: 978-1-4917-7068-9 (e)

Library of Congress Control Number: 2015909565

Print information available on the last page.

iUniverse rev. date: 08/25/2015

CONTENTS

ACKNOWLEDGMENTS

First, being of the utmost importance, I thank my Lord and Savior, Jesus Christ, because without his mercy and grace set upon me, I know these accomplishments would not exist. My Lord and Savior, Jesus Christ, has kept his hands on me with his ever-so-shining bright light at my feet, which has led me appropriately down my life's path. It is clear his guidance put me where I am today without having to search for tomorrow. My faith, strengthened through his love and prayer every morning and every night, and accommodated by his wisdom, knowledge, and understanding affixed to my heart, mind, body, and soul, guided me to communicate my study as intentional instruction in this form of current literature and research so that all could learn and benefit.

I met several professors on my road to further achievement at Walden University who all deserve recognition. I am very fortunate to have the opportunity to thank my professors and classmates at Walden University. I'd also like to thank my mother, Bessie Edison; father; brother; sisters; and friends for their tireless support and team spirit, which kept me stimulated and excited all the way through my comprehensive management masters science leadership (MMSL) journey.

I must acknowledge my first point of contact when I enrolled in Walden University, Arlene Starr, enrollment adviser at the School of Management and Technology, Richard W. Riley College of Education and Leadership. My path, similar to hers and so many others', was made possible by the founders of Walden University, Bernie and Rita Turner, and their steadfast diligence and commitment to make a way for future adult graduate students. Arlene's knowledge and understanding of adult students' academic desires allowed her to sense what I needed to be exposed as I made the critical decision of which institution would further my education. One of the top regional online-accredited universities in America presented the mission statement heard throughout the nation. Simply stated, my decision to put my trust in "a higher degree" and "a higher purpose"—Walden's motto—really set the stage and proved that their path unequivocally was the one for me to take for extraordinary academic achievement.

In addition, thank you to Ray Samson, Center for Personal and Professional Development—Virtual Education Center (VEC), Oceana Naval Base, Dam Neck Annex, Virginia Beach, Virginia. He invested his interest in my academic requirements and ensured all the i's were dotted and all the t's were crossed on important documents like tuition-assistance applications and vouchers submitted through the navy campus, the VEC, and Walden University registrar and admissions departments. Thanks also to everyone working endless days and hours at the Department of Veteran Affairs, Veterans Administration Educational Benefits Office, for their timely processing of my Montgomery and Post-9/11 GI Bills, which provided the funds for my Walden University tuition, books, and fees.

During the course of my learning experience, a pure blessing found me by way of having the opportunity to create a peer group with Walden University expertise and experience, which consisted of a wide range of professional and personal leadership disciplines and techniques. I owe a ton of gratitude to all the professors who had a hand in my academic and professional development at Walden University.

I also thank Dr. David Morton for sharing his inspirational knowledge about the value of cultural experiences and embracing leadership excellence. I'd like to thank Dr. Pettis Perry for sharing his unique method of learning disciplines in the form of his course survival guide, and for instilling in me the belief to trust in the principles of diversity, which connected me with my classmates, their perspectives and cultures, and the mission of Walden University. His practices motivated me to create an intellectual framework to success, which helped me develop and better communicate solutions in my academic, personal, and professional environments.

In addition, thank you to Dr. Cherif Sidialicherif for sharing his thorough knowledge and providing valuable information about the power of cultural intelligence and the challenges of global leadership. He served as my personal guide through the course and increased my awareness of different leadership styles, improving my adaptability and flexibility skills to become a better overall leader. Thanks also to Dr. Gordon McLean for providing his extensive knowledge about research strategies for leaders and paradigms, how to deal with social changes, and the different models of leadership, which expanded my knowledge base and situational awareness about the depths and expectations of leadership as a Walden University graduate student and in society.

Thank you to Dr. Maria Minor for sharing her extensive knowledge about the learning organization and how to preserve the excellence of and commitment to leadership, trust, and integrity, which promotes internal and external growth in not only the learning organization but in my working environment. I also owe a great deal of gratitude to Dr. Marilyn Dickey, who was inspirational and extremely helpful. She offered priceless assistance as a professor, providing constructive feedback and support that raised my innovative and technology leadership skill sets and prepared me for the next level of leading in any organizational environment, academically and professionally.

I also convey my gratitude to Dr. David Thornton for making available his superb instruction and guidance in the course of strategies for advancing in innovation, technology, and strategic management in the workforce. I benefitted from the principles he demonstrated, which proved to be his blueprint to solutions and directions to achievement, by sharing those beliefs with my peers and colleagues. This in turn made me a better leader, innovator, and facilitator of technology in my organizational learning environment.

I extend my thank-you to Dr. Padma Viswanathan for sharing his experience in the course of advanced technologies, management of innovation, and management styles, which consisted of numerous stimulating discussions that helped me understand how I could be a greater contributor and leader in the innovation and technology arena.

Dr. Marilys Taylor opened and closed the chapters of my academic achievements, leaving me to fill in the middle. Dr. Taylor revealed the leadership traits and the value of understanding how to be a great leader. Her willingness to stay involved in my studies by providing constructive feedback and encouragement kept me motivated, which contributed enormously to my academic success.

Dr. Taylor brilliantly guided me with an influential hand in every move of my learning experience. Her influence was deeply rooted in me from the start of my graduate studies through its final destination, my comprehensive capstone research project. Her expertise and encouragement throughout this course were phenomenal and set the mark for academic and professional leadership and commitment at the highest institutional level for not only me but also the entire MMSL class.

At last, and most especially, I thank my amazing and supportive wife, Taniko, a true blessing for her calm willingness to endure and her loving spirit, which kept me even more motivated over the last two years of my graduate school studies. The academic journey I elected to take and merge with the duties and responsibilities of continuous service to the United States in twenty-six years of active duty naval service added to the already intense challenges and high operational tempo in our lives, which included two wars. Taniko was simply the best wife on the planet, demonstrating unquestioned devotion, loyalty, trust, steadfast commitment, and unconditional love for me and our unified beliefs instilled in us by God Almighty to continue to improve ourselves.

ABSTRACT

This research project paper explores, discusses, and examines the social impact of organ donation and transplantation processes and procedures that affect donors, recipients, family members, and health and medical researchers. A factor included in the research with an immediate effect on the organ donation and transplantation process is shortages of donors. Claims presented state that the primary reason for shortage of donors nationally and globally is a lack of education and information about organ donation and transplantation, which would allow potential donors to make informed decisions. In addition, some organizations have offered incentives and rewards to donors if they volunteer their organs to the waiting list. However, once declared brain-dead, the processes and procedures take a different course, as power nations like the United Kingdom and the United States of America have their own viewpoints when determining terminology and protocols. Most important is a look at the biomedical concerns that have come to the forefront because of pathopsychological changes that create other major considerations. Also discussed is the role that families play in overriding loved ones' expressed wishes to be donors. Required counseling for recipients, donors, and families has been developed in some areas. It includes health and medical researchers working in the organ donation and transplantation industry.

INTRODUCTION

National and global crises exist around inconsistencies in the organ donation and transplantation health and medical industry. The following chapters from my research show factors attributing to the current situation of organ donation and transplantation and prove there are major challenges that require immediate attention.

Organ donation and transplantation are a global concern, with different viewpoints questioned and unanswered by religions, governments, and the people. Concerns challenge the health and medical industry regarding organ donation and major transplantation. Above all, global supply and demand is critically unbalanced, and health and medical researchers are desperately trying to figure out ways to mitigate this crisis. Hearts, kidneys, lungs, livers, and pancreases are at the very top of the global waiting list. Furthermore, the gap between supply and demand is constantly increasing, with a growing recipient waiting list and a stalled donor acquisition list.

More contributing factors to the unbalanced supply and demand are educational. People are not equipped with the information needed to make a decision in favor of organ donation and transplantation. A major challenge is the lack of national and global educational programs to teach the public about the importance of organ donation and transplantation. The shortage of education available to the public about organ donation and transplantation processes and procedures adversely affects every society on the planet. Statistics show the majority of the uneducated support a lifesaving initiative. This negatively influences all other conditions and concerns. My findings prove the processes and procedures have become overwhelming severe nationally and globally because of biased behavior and foul play by some organizations, and the absence of protocols that support established ethics to guard against breaking the rules.

The resources utilized for this research consist of the following criteria, which covers eligibility of organ donors, the donor-recipient authorization process, agencies authorized for procurement, regulations for prioritizing candidates, age differences, gender distinction, quality, quantity, and at what level diversity influences the decision making as far as global continuity and discretion. The focus is on the entire scope of what, when, where, how, and why it takes place in the health and medical world of organ donation and transplantation.

My testable predictions are based on innovative ideals and technological disciplines incorporated with the practices acquired through extensive study in leadership. This prepared me academically and professionally to ascertain vital health and medical data about organ donation, transplantation, and their effects on the public. Resources used consisted of databases from the Walden University library, journal articles, books, magazines, newspapers, websites, audio and video media, and the human factor. The ultimate task is to inform communities and societies on a global scale of the importance of supporting organ donation and transplantation if they so desire. Volunteering to donate an organ is not mandatory. However, if the results of the process are clearly stated and understood by administrators and participants, I believe a gradual balance between donations and need will occur.

Subsequent steps include spreading this knowledge at a national level and then submitting to the global network an analysis and discussion points to recommend practice guidelines for transplant physicians, primary-care providers, health-care planners, and all those concerned about the well-being of the live organ donor (http://europepmc.org/abstract/MED/11187711/reload=0;jsessionid=PgDewPe5O4jfxn4ZIpLW.20). Any source permitting legal and ethical procurement has the right to be recognized as a global team player in support of the crisis.

Before we look at how to alleviate the problem, we have to put the problem in context.

CHAPTER 1
CONTEXT

This context statement begins with information about an analysis developed through extensive research. Furthermore, based on the nature and sensitivity of the organ donor process surrounding this research project, my objective is on course to educate people about the world of organ donors. Examples provided in this discussion begin a process of pass, understand, and accept knowledge of the steps and procedures that include various levels of the processes ascending or descending in an event chain working order. Included in the research are concepts based on community change context and how it interrelates to the objective set forth, which "permits the introduction of new elements into the theoretical concepts of leadership and offers a different perspective on leadership for change, such as power and empowerment" (Hickman 2010, 121). Hickman also provided awareness to understanding that "change agents turn to their own resources to conduct participatory action research (PAR)" (121). In this case, however, it resides in the medical arena of organ donors.

A long time ago there were scientists, physicians, surgeons, authors, and curiosity about the body's organs and what happens to them once human beings enter that final stage of life. Over the centuries, organ donors and transplants have become significantly synonymous, in that one does not exist without the other. Let me share a case and point provided by Armitage, Tullo, and Larkin (2006).

When Austrian physician Eduard Zirm transplanted the corneas of an eleven-year-old boy to a day laborer, Alois Glogar, who had recently become blind in an accident while slaking lime, on December 7, 1905, he made a breakthrough in the science of organ transplantation. (as cited in Sims 2010, 10)

Even before Eduard Zirm exploration into anatomy, in the "1700s, as physicians began to learn about the marks that pathologies left on bodies, performing autopsies became increasingly important in their education" (Baker and Hargreaves 2001, 1–42) and became the most ethical medical method in analyzing, preserving, and transferring body organs.

Researchers began experimenting with organ transplantation in animals and humans in the eighteenth century. Over the years, scientists experienced many failures, but by the mid-twentieth century, successful organ transplants had been performed. Transplants of kidneys, livers, hearts, lungs, pancreases, and small bowels are now an accepted part of medical treatment. Bone marrow transplants save lives and corneal transplants restore sight. Medical miracles happen every day (http://www.schooleymitchell. com/english/charity/och_history.php).

Organ donations are right in the thick of medical miracles. I believe miracles, including medical ones, have a direct connection to spiritualism, an exciting science yet still a natural, human wonder. Society's unanswered questions can assist in saving the few, meaning those who are fortunate enough to obtain a needed transplant, if general awareness is in place. However, I provide a pathway to strength and courage toward entering the unknown. In support of this, Marquardt (2005) asserted that "courage includes the willingness to ask questions that might challenge— even break up—current perceptions and patterns" (53) about the analysis of the current processes of and procedures involved in organ donation. Thus, the questions we ask will lead to eventually attaining the right answers.

CHAPTER 2
CASE UNDER STUDY

Health and medical research organizations act as catalysts in the structure and development of the organ donor organizational processes, rules, and regulations by adjusting the uniform movement and applications of complex science to virtual medical technology and terminology. According to Howard, Cornell, and Cochran (2012), "the concept of transplantation, taking parts from one animal or person and putting them into another animal or person, is ancient, thus the development of organ transplantation brought on the need for a source of organs" (6). The need for human organs is rapidly increasing every year based on the National Network of Organ Donors (NNOD), which stated, "the statistics are staggering and the statistics are heartbreaking. More than 113,000 people are currently on UNOS' (United Network for Organ Sharing) transplant waiting list, and the number of people who die waiting for transplants continues to grow: from 10 people each day in 1990, to 14 a day in 1996, to 19 today" (http://www.thenationalnetworkoforgandonors.org/). Howard et al. (2012) indicated, "this need for organs to satisfy the great demand led to specialized organizations to identify deceased donors, manage them until recovery occurred, and to notify transplant centers that organs were available for their patients" (6). Furlow (2012) pointed out the numbers are alarming: "Thousands of Americans die each year awaiting donated hearts, lungs, kidneys, and pancreata—victims of shortages in donated organs. Because organ degradation begins soon after brain death ensues, even in the presence of a heartbeat, the central paradox of organ transplantation medicine has been described as 'the need for both a living body and a dead donor'" (371). Sims (2010) noted, "In 1984, the United States government passed the National Organ Transplant Act (NOTA), and this act affected organ transplants in many significant ways" (11).

During these developments, Howard et al. (2012) said,

> because of the shortage of organs relative to the demand, lack of a unified organ allocation system, the perception that organs are a national resource and should be governed by national regulations, and to improve results of organ procurement organizations and transplant centers, the federal government has regulated virtually all phases of organ procurement and transplantation. (6)

Sims (2010) tells us:

- First of all, it made it illegal to buy or sell organs in the United States.
- Secondly, a large, non-profit organization called the United Network for Organ Sharing (UNOS) was founded.
- Third, this organization was created to oversee several regional nonprofit organizations called Organ Procurement Organizations (OPOs). (11)

"In 1998, the act was amended and hospitals were required to contact OPOs when possible organ donors died or were near death" (Sims 2010, 11).

With organ donations being launched at a time when medical science was thirsting for more, monitoring of ethical behavior throughout these organizations was probably under strict observation by all sides when the conversation turned to near death or patients who would possibly die soon. To me, this has to be one of the most complex medical environments to practice in. Those individuals must rely more on the findings within their subconsciouses. For example, "when an organ that has potential for donation becomes available, the hospital gives it to an OPO, which matches the organ with the most deserving recipient" (Sims 2010, 11). Diethelm (1990) stated, "The preliminary criteria that UNOS's system uses to match organs with possible recipients are organ type, organ size, and blood type" (as cited in Sims 2010, 11).

The demand created from the new technologies set in motion by the new, innovative studies behind the organ donation process expanded with more organizations and with more by-laws that incorporated themselves within the existing guidance. In moving forward, Doig and Rocker (2003) reported, "the increasing gap between numbers of individuals awaiting organ replacement surgery and the supply of organs available for transplant underpins attempts to increase the number of organs available" (1,069). This led to the creation of "one practice, used in other countries that is the recovery of organs from non-heart-beating organ donors (NHBD)" (Doig and Rocker 2003, 1,069).

There are several ethical debates surrounding organ donor processes and procedures, because the different organizations with a hand in acquisitions dig deeper and deeper for individual control. For instance, Sims (2010) determined one "ethical dilemma involving the redefinition of death and organ transplants hinges on the fact that a healthy human being could donate one kidney and still live normally with one functioning kidney" (10). On the other hand, Doig and Rocker (2003) noted the following analysis.

> NHBD protocols have been established in many countries including the United States. Despite numerous publications, and extensive debate in the literature, significant ethical issues remain unresolved in the retrieval of organs from donors that have died from cessation of cardiac activity. The ethical concerns primarily arise in the determination of

death, the tension between the time constraints on recovering organs viable for transplantation, and procedures to enhance organ viability. (1,069)

The benefits of today's new technology were paved through such actions as those noted by Howard et al. (2012), which stated,

The first use of a kidney for transplantation in the modern era of transplantation occurred in 1947, when Dr. David Hume transplanted a kidney from someone who had died (cardiac death) into a young woman with postpartum renal failure. The renal artery and vein were sutured to the brachial vessels and a cutaneous ureterostomy was constructed. The kidney functioned until the patient's own kidneys recovered. (7)

This was a miracle for the time. This phenomenon attracted the curiosity of new organizations, seeking to venture into the wealth of organ donation and transplantation, ultimately leading to more laws and more regulations. Moreover, a step in the right direction was created that leaned heavily toward a waiting list for every transplantable organ used within the organ donation centers. More information about the organ donor waiting list process and procedures is covered later.

Check this assertion based on "the rationale behind using NHBD which includes:

1) the NHBD was the major source of organs for transplantation prior to the development and adoption of brain death criteria, and remains so in countries, e.g., Japan, where the concept of "brain death" has only recently been adopted in legislation, but has yet to be widely accepted by the general populace;

2) the recovery of organs from NHBD does not violate the ethical principle of the "dead donor" rule (see below); and

3) the determination of death by cardiopulmonary criteria is far more common; therefore, the pool of potential donors would include a larger group of patients, not only those patients dying from catastrophic brain injury" (Doig and Rocker 2003, 1,070)

According to Sims (2010), however, "the best candidates to donate hearts to those in need were patients that were brain dead, on life support, but had healthy hearts" (Sims 2010, 10). The amazement to this case study developed "before the Ad Hoc Committee's ruling, surgeons had to wait in frustration for a patient to be ruled dead before taking the heart, which seriously minimized its effectiveness in the recipient's body" (Sims 2010, 10–11). Sims noted that this "new definition of death allowed surgeons to keep irreversibly comatose patients on life support while their hearts were removed so to ensure the heart would not be ruined" (11).

Keep in mind the medical science that influenced the health and medical community in honor of the organ donor was never a sweet science but has become a global, advancing science, with worldwide interest in procurement. Speaking of global procurement, legitimate organizations, communities, and centers also combat the adversities created by negative challenges from organ trafficking and the impact it has placed on donors and recipients.

Furthermore, organized crime has a vested interest in organ donations and transplantation. Black market trades and other illegal organizations have also become more widespread in the organ transplantation arena, with their hands deep in buying and selling organs to the highest bidders. In the upcoming chapters, I discuss how illegal organ traffickers break restrictions and regulations, compromising the availability of healthy organs to those in need but without the means to purchase them from alternative sources.

Table 2.1 Organ Procurement and Transplantation
Network Wait List Data (a)

Organ Type	No. Patients on Wait List for Donated Organ
All	112 648
Kidneys	90 542
Liver	16 035
Pancreas	1361
Kidney and pancreas	2205
Heart	3138
Lung	1775
Intestine	264
Heart and lung	67
(a) Data current as of January 19, 2012. Source: http://optn.transplant.gov/data, Furlow, 2012, p. 372; Edison, 2013.	

The numbers tell the story. According to Furlow (2012), more than "112,648 people in the United States were awaiting lifesaving organ donations as of January 2012. It is estimated that more than 4,000 new patients are added to the national waiting list each month" (371).

Historically, Furlow (2012) noted the following.

> Archeological evidence suggests surgical bone grafts may have been attempted thousands of years ago. Although almost certainly mythological, 5000-year-old Hindu texts describe the use of skin autografts (i.e., tissue or organ grafts transplanted into a recipient from the same donor or a genetically identical donor) from patients' buttocks and chins to reconstruct their noses cut off as punishment. (372)

Hickman (2010) asked, "So how does a relatively powerless and underrepresented group of people organize to effectively protect their community against the threat of an environmental hazard?" (130). How do they protect against unpredictable occurrences not in favor of the concepts of change? In this context, "the answer entails familiar aspects of theoretical concepts of leadership—values, adaptive work, leadership without authority, and the common and distinguishing elements of leadership" (Hickman 2010, 130). This section of research and analysis is a direct reflection of how long global organizations and communities have been dealing with the dynamics of the organ donor process, whether voluntarily or involuntarily. Health and medical science evolving around organ donations has elevated universally for the sake of humanity.

CHAPTER 3

STATEMENT OF THE PROBLEM

The organ donation and transplantation process has proven to save lives. Many people have benefited from the health and medical research conducted to establish legitimate programs and organizations supporting people who need the services. Despite the process's success, there are difficulties.

In my research I found mixed emotions concerning the organ donor process, especially in the donor family. Those emotions include anxiety, frustration, failure, pain, joy, and happiness. Individuals, families, and friends must deal with these emotions during what can be a long, difficult decision-making process.

My research determined the number-one problem with the organ donation and transplantation processes and procedures falls on supply and demand. Demand far outweighs the supply of organs available for transplant. This means many people die waiting for lifesaving transplants.

According to Galandiuk and Sterioff (2005), "The current system for procuring and distributing organs to patients in need has failed despite pertinacious efforts to keep up with demand" (320). Furthermore, "transplant physicians and surgeons have compounded the problem by expanding the criteria for transplantation beyond the original restrictions on age, comorbidities, and systemic disease" (320).

Physicians and nonphysicians are attracted to the organ donation enterprise. Why is this so important in the arena of transplantation? When it comes to loved ones, desperation comes in to play, and the visions of some recipients, families, and organizations get a little cloudy, leading them to become fixated on seeking any means necessary to resolve their current situation. For example, "the need for engaging non-physicians in the requesting process is further dictated by the fact that most physicians have never asked a family for an organ donation, even though they may refer patients with organ failure to transplant centers" (Galandiuk and Sterioff 2005, 320).

Information gathered from the National Network of Organ Donors website provided the following assertion.

> The problem isn't that people don't want to donate organs or even that they don't sign up to become donors. It is that currently, the health care and legal systems do not ensure that a person's wishes regarding organ donation are honored. Even if you sign a donor card or the back of your driver's license, if your family does not give its approval, the hospital will not procure your organs—in spite of your prior written consent. The National Network of Organ Donors believes that signing a legal document should guarantee, without exception, that your wishes are met (http://www.thenationalnetworkoforgandonors.org/about.html), but to say the least, even after a person has entered the final stages of life, family approval still has to be met, regardless. With all the discussion going on about organ donation and transplantation, the entire process should not be taken for granted. Warren (1992) reminds us of a true case and point that families experience attributed to the organ donor

national situation: The problem was driven home dramatically last week when a 26-year-old Burbank woman died 30 hours after doctors at Cedars-Sinai Medical Center transplanted a pig's liver into her body until they could locate a human liver. The crux of the problem is not Americans' unwillingness to become donors. Opinion polls consistently show 60% to 70% of Americans support donation and would donate the organs of a family member if asked. (3)

After reading the case, you must ask yourself about the role of health and medical organizations in procuring a supply of animal organs. Although those organs went through rigorous examinations, were studied and then assumed to work, was it ethical to use the organs in human beings? This may carry over as a direct reflection on the perception of evolution. In a world of division, some, even scientists and innovators today, believe humans evolved from the ape, and since the history of technology has gravitated to perpetuate the subconscious to the point that proven health and medical research dictates direction in critical decision making, the result is why not? Galandiuk and Sterioff (2005) stated, "use of animals in research, animal organs for transplantation, and embryonic stem cell research are bellwether subjects, as is the recent passage of Proposition 71 in California, which supports funding for stem cell research" (320). California's Proposition 71 also supports animal transplantation as a human organ substitute. This is a completely different strategy to balancing the overwhelming limited supply of organs and the huge demand.

According to Warren (1992), the issue also involves the donation process itself. "The problem lies within the system and a combination of factors that have led experts to understand that the potential donor pool is considerably smaller than once thought" (3). In addition, the organ donor processes and procedures are more complex than what meets the eye. Adding more insult to injury, this current research and analysis regarding organ shortfalls finds global organizations that should be supporting the cause are searching for an independent advantage. Kierans and Cooper (2011) stated, "Low rates of organ donation among what are routinely referred to in healthcare domains as 'black and minority ethnic' (BME) 'communities' (here denoting people of African, Caribbean and South Asian backgrounds) are a problem that emerges within the professional matrix of UK transplant medicine and the organization of the health service to which it connects" (11).

Many recipients are led to believe what Warren (1992) processed: "Part of the problem is caused by a shrinking donor pool. Ten years ago, the federal Centers for Disease Control estimated that the potential number of eligible donors per year ranged from 13,750 to 29,000. Recent studies indicate that those figures are much too optimistic" (1).

Roger Evans (1992) "projects the potential donor supply to be between 6,900 and 10,700 annually, and places the most 'realistic estimate of potential donors at 7,300 each year, based on a 53% to 68% rate of consent to donate'" (as cited in Warren 1992, 1).

Individuals and families waiting for the call that a donor match is available could be filled with anxiety, pressure, and stress. Shah and Bhosale (2006) made an assessment based on India: "In a developing country like ours, slow growth of organ transplantation is due to high costs involved, lack of facilities in government hospitals, non-availability of a suitable donor from the family and lack of well-developed cadaver programs" (29). India isn't alone. Kierans and Cooper (2011) report, "access to suitable organs for transplant in the UK has been restricted by an explicit orientation towards cadaveric donation and an 'opt-in' system of participation" (12). These findings have potential global interest.

Biological effects also contribute to lack of organ donations. Davies (2006) determined that "for anyone classified as a 'BME' patient, these structural constraints on organ viability have been compounded by allocation policies that favor blood group and tissue, or HLA (human leukocyte antigen), matching" (as cited in Kierans and Cooper 2011, 12). The HLA is a gene product of the major histocompatibility complex. These antigens have a strong influence on human allotransplantation, transfusions in refractory patients, and certain disease associations (http://medical-dictionary.thefreedictionary.com/human+leukocyte+antigen). Moreover, it is the type of molecule found on the surface of most cells in the body. HLAs play an important part in the body's immune response to foreign substances. They make up a person's tissue type. HLA tests are done before a donor stem-cell or organ transplant to find out if donor and recipient tissues match (http://www.cancer.gov/dictionary?cdrid=386210). These tests are vital and a standard health and medical practice in organ and tissue transplants. They should never be taken lightly despite a family's urgency to receive an organ donation.

Whenever there is a large discrepancy between supply and demand, there will be people with unorthodox ideas for solving the problem. Warren (1992) noted, "Lloyd Cohen, a Chicago lawyer, advocates creating a market system in cadaveric transplant organs and tissues. Cohen supports establishing a 'futures market' that would allow individuals to 'contract for the sale of their body tissue for delivery after their death'" (10). In my opinion, this practice creates an independent marketplace for body organs. In addition, "In Cohen's rather complicated system, once an enrolled person's organs are recovered and transplanted after his death, 'a payment in the range of $5,000 for each major organ and lesser amounts for minor tissues would be made to the donor's estate or designee'" (Warren 1992, 10). One has to wonder whether insurance companies, many of whom hesitate to cover all expenses of traditional donation, would cover these costs.

The following is a review of the basic requirements for organ donation and transplantation.

Successful Organ Donation Requires

- Identification of potential organ donor
- Determination and certification of brain death
- Consent to organ donation from the family
- Diagnosis and management of organ donor problems

- Organ retrieval and transplantation (Shah and Bhosale 2006, 29)

Another factor to consider in the organ donation and transplantation process is the family. We must remember organ donation and transplantation are sensitive and delicate matters. The family of the recipient carries a huge burden on its shoulders when caring for the family recipient. If the donor is deceased, one must keep in mind that the family is facing a loss, often under tragic circumstances. If the organ is coming from a living donor, his or her family—as well as the donor—likely feels anxious about the possible dangers of the surgery.

Interviewing and counseling with compassion are proven practices that need to be applied during and after the waiting period. According to Shaw (2011), "In the case of organ donor family members and transplant recipients it is arguably the absence of discussion around questions of shared intercorporeality between anonymous donors and recipients in the donation and transplantation context that produces anxiety" (63).

Hockey (2007) provided her perspective of the problem as "taken for granted the assumption about doing research in the field of death and dying is that this is a particularly sensitive area to work in and researchers need to take extra care to ensure the emotional and psychic safety of research participants, as well as monitor and manage their own research experiences" (as cited in Shaw 2011, 63). I impress on researchers to carry out these duties with the best interests of the recipients and family members—donor and recipient families—in mind. Shaw (2011) says, "This often requires researchers to provide contact details of relevant counselors, therapists or hotlines for welfare agencies on participant information sheets in case of interviewees' distress during or after a standard interview" (62). During this third-party assessment, Shaw reminds us that "organ transfer also raises a number of ethical and emotional issues, especially in discussions around anonymity protocol and in relation to the invisible but tangible presence of shared corporeality in the course of organ transfer" (62).

There is one problem left to research and analyze: the truth about global black marketing of human organs. The crime entails more than illegally selling human organs. Associated kidnapping and human trafficking means more laws being broken. I believe this is all based on who has the money, which equates to who's the highest bidder. As noted by Scheper-Hughes (2003), "In all, we have begun to map the routes and the international medical and financial connections that make possible the new traffic in human beings, a veritable slave trade that can bring together parties from three or more countries" (1,645). I believe much of this trafficking involves organized crime in the buying and selling of high-stakes human body organs and transplantation.

Scheper-Hughes (2003) reports, "Brokers in Brooklyn, New York, posing as a non-profit organization, traffic in Russian immigrants to service foreign patients from Israel who are transplanted in some of the best medical facilities on the east coast of the USA" (1,646). In addition to that deception, "Wealthy Palestinians travel to Iraq where they can buy a kidney from poor Arabs coming from Jordan" (1,646). More often than not, "the circulation of kidneys follows established routes of capital from South to North, from East to West, from poorer to more affluent bodies, from black and brown bodies to white ones, and from female to male or from poor, low status men to more affluent men" (1,645). In what may be a surprise, Scheper-Hughes found, "women are rarely the recipients of purchased organs anywhere in the world" (1,645). However, Scheper-Hughes discovery does not deter or slow down the program.

Warren (1992) reported this black-market scenario: "Why should the donor receive $1,000 for agreeing to donate his or her organs in anticipation of death? Pellegrino argues. 'What will keep the price from escalating if an insufficient number of organs are procured? ... A black market of covert payments exceeding the going rate is certain to rise'" (12).

16

The results of a UNOS survey about compensation and organ transplantation published in 1991 were alarming (See table 3.1).

Table 3.1 "Public Attitudes about Financial Incentives

Percentage	Results
52%	Favored financial or some other type of compensation
22%	Opposed to any compensation
5%	Abuse the system
2%	Lead to Black Market" (Warren, 1992, p. 13; Edison, 2013)

Scheper-Hughes (2003) reported, "From an exclusively market oriented supply and demand perspective—one that is obviously dominant today—the problem of black markets in human organs can best be solved by regulation rather than by prohibition" (1,646). For example, "National regulatory programs—such as the Kid-Net program (modeled after commercial blood banks), which is currently being considered in the Philippines—would still have to compete with international black markets, which adjust the local value of kidneys according to consumer prejudices (1,647)."

The fact of the matter is displayed as a result of current trends.

> In today's global market an Indian or an African kidney fetches as little as $1,000, a Filipino kidney can get $1,300, a Moldovan or Romanian kidney yields $2,700, whereas a Turkish or an urban Peruvian kidney can command up to $10,000 or more and sellers in the USA can receive up to $30,000, thus putting a market price on body parts—even a fair one—exploits the desperation of the poor, the mentally weak, and dependent classes (Scheper-Hughes 2003, 1,647).

CHAPTER 4

RESEARCH ISSUES

The previous three chapters stated the issues included in this research project. All arouse curiosity and are thought provoking, complicated, and challenging. To increase the possibility I will be able to make additional discoveries revolving around organ donation and transplantation, I have limited my research to two issues.

The risk of no-holds-barred procurement outweighs ethical guidelines the world must follow. If these guidelines are followed, the procurement process could still be successful. Historically and globally, however, the entire process has produced a by-product—a profitable market for human body organs.

I find it amazing that health and medical research is not completely at its best. While advancements have been made in organ and tissue transplantation, there are areas that can be expanded, possibly making more organs available for transplantation.

Research Issue #1

> Is global organ shortage really due to families nullifying the expressed desire of their loved ones to donate their organs after death?

The organ donor and transplantation process across the world grows more uncertain because donors, recipients, and families lack education about the procedural steps. Information provided by health and medical agencies and organizations is generic and does not take into account information specific individuals may need to make a well-informed decision. Families involved in the process must know they and their loved ones are receiving the attention they need. This develops trust in the efforts of those on the organ procurement and transplant team, which can help smooth the transition. Families can then have the confidence they made the right decisions. Sque et al. (2008) stated, "Relatives of potential deceased donors remain critical links in maintaining organ supply, as organ donation is normally discussed with them and their support, agreement or lack of objection sought before donation takes place ... an understanding of what motivates families to agree or decline donation is therefore essential to maximize organ availability" (134–135). However, Burroughs et al. (1998) stated, "unfortunately, there are few studies of how families who decline donation view their decisions or experience bereavement" (as cited in Sque et al. 2008, 136). Hence, "greater understanding is therefore needed about the decision-making process that motivates families of potential deceased organ donors to decline donation and how they construe their decision-making experience" (Sque et al. 2008, 136).

Table 4.1 Educational Factors of Influence and Declination, illustrates the thoughts behind the decision-making process.

Factors of Influence	Factors of Declination
"Knowledge of the deceased's wishes, particularly, if these had been discussed with the family, or the family believed that the person would have agreed to or declined donation	Divisions within the family about the decision.
Not understanding the concept of death certified by brain-based, neurological criteria.	'Non-white' ethnicity.

19

Not wanting surgery to the body, fearing that the body would be disfigured.	Dissatisfaction with the quality of care the deceased and family received in hospital.
Feeling that the deceased had suffered enough.	Perceptions of surprise, pressure, or harassment about donation decisions. Untimely information. Individual needs not being addressed. Feelings about not coping with the decision and wanting to be present when the ventilator was switched off."

Source: Sque et al. 2008, 135; Edison 2013.

Interviews were conducted by intensive care units that provided other reasons why families declined organ donation from deceased love ones. Here are the results from those interviews.

- The circumstances leading up to the death of their relative.
- Their experiences in hospital.
- Their views about the care that was provided both for the sick relative and for the family.
- Their experience of being informed about the death of the relative and any discussion about brain-stem death and organ donation.
- How they made the decision not to donate.
- Their reasons for not donating.
- Any impact the decision had.
- Any particular bereavement needs they felt they had and the type and quality of bereavement care offered. (Sque et al. 2008, 137)

Organ donation and transplantation decisions come down to what you really know and what you are asked to believe in. If information about the process isn't clear, you cannot blame families for what they do not know. Again, educate families on the entire process of organ donation and transplantation. Sque et al. (2008) stated, "A lack of knowledge—some participants lacked information about what the process of organ donation actually involved" (139).

Those involved in the process must be able to answer all questions families have. Some are easier to answer than others, of course. I believe some families asked questions like "Is the deceased safe?" Despite the emotional circumstances surrounding the death of their relatives, if families can make a well-informed decision, they may find solace knowing they and their loved ones have helped others.

Research Issue #2

> With twenty-first-century advancements in leadership, innovation, and technology in the health and medical industry, what options are available to eliminate the use of animal organs in humans?

The most logical answer to research issue 2 is to keep it at the drawing board, meaning continue to build on those advancements and technologies in the health and medical industry, no matter how long it takes. Humankind's impatience to keep up with organ demand takes the organ and transplant process on a course of no looking back, as advancements are made in transplanting animal organs and tissues in humans. O'Neill (2006) stated, "The transplantation of animal organs and tissues into humans raises a number of social, ethical, moral, and political issues, many of which have yet to be fully resolved" (211).

Despite these issues, the latest medical technology involves xenotransplantation. According to Mortier et al. (2004), "xenotransplantation is the practice of transplanting, implanting, or infusing cells, tissues, or organs from one species to another" (as cited in O'Neill 2006, 211). In support of this medical technology, Rosenkrantz (1996) stated, "pig skin has been used for over 20 years to treat burns victims, heart valves from pigs have been used to replace damaged human valves, and pig cell islets are used in the manufacture of insulin for diabetics" (as cited in O'Neill 2006, 223). Deschamps et al. (2005) stated, "There is a well-documented history of attempts at clinical xenotransplantation between different animal species" (213). O'Neill (2006) indicated, "It was not until the 1960s that concerted efforts were made to transplant animal organs into human patients" (213). Thus, history was made.

Further research has led to the discovery "of the various attempts at transplanting the organs of an animal into a human, two instances in particular warrant close consideration" (O'Neill 2006, 213). Deschamps et al. (2005) pointed out, "The first occurred on October 26, 1984, at the Loma Linda University Hospital, California, where Dr. Leonard Bailey transplanted a baboon heart into a newborn girl" (as cited in O'Neill 2006, 213). Although the procedure appeared encouraging, "the 15-day-old infant was dying of hypo plastic left-heart syndrome and had no chance of surviving without a transplant." Sadly, "the girl died 21 days post-operation and became known as 'the Baby Fae case,' which attracted considerable media attention and the public became transfixed by the real possibility of neonatal cardiac transplantation" (213).

This discovery led to another. Johnston (1991) pointed out, "it also created awareness of the demand for, and lack of, newborn human organs, a situation not previously publicized, as well as awareness of the potential benefits of organ transplantation during neonatal life" (as cited in O'Neill 2006, 213).

The growing interest in cross-species transplantations found more parties getting involved that were concerned with the ethics of these experiments. The Nuffield Council on Bioethics (1996) provided the following statement.

> Animal-to-human transplantation: The ethics of xenotransplantation, had also recommended that an advisory committee on xenotransplantation be established for the purpose of 'assessing the potential public health risk from infectious organisms of

animals, establishing the essential precautionary measures prior to any clinical human trials, and protecting the interests of the patients who receive xenografts.' (as cited in O'Neill 2006, 218)

Even if there were definitive alternatives to animal-human organ transplantation, it may be an afterthought. This is because of the marketplace and the growing need to fill shortages in worldwide organ donation supply. O'Neill (2006) stated, "Patients who are financially impoverished, and for whom the cost of a human organ transplant was prohibitive, may also find xenotransplantation an attractive proposition." Keep in mind that "the characteristic common to these potential patients is their vulnerability, brought about by the unlikelihood of them obtaining a suitable human organ" (224).

In conclusion, the following assessment is provided.

> Despite consistent media reports, xenotransplantation is not as developed as is commonly believed. An enormous amount of research has still to be carried out before the practice becomes a reality. However, it may be pointless expending huge amounts of money, energy, and time on such research if society, in general, is unwilling to accept the transplantation of animal organs. While medical researchers may be able to overcome problems associated with the biological rejection of animal organs by the human immune system, the insurmountable problem may be rejection of xenotransplantation by society. (O'Neill 2006, 228).

I believe in this arena, the option of choice is heavily weighed when deliberating what the medical research industry has invested and brought to the table. Meaning that, families could be convinced in these particular cases of what is needed, what is right versus what is wrong. The greater value equals a huge possibility of saving and extending a loved one's life, which revolves around transplantation, implantation, or infusion of resources from a nonhuman species to a recipient human species. In addition, has thought gone into the rights of the nonhuman species and at what cost? Nonetheless, is there a populace 100 percent onboard with xenotransplantation?

CHAPTER 5
METHODS

M y research and analysis methods included recorded interviews, observations, and surveys. The methods varied for each concern but provide sound, innovative solutions for the crisis created by a lack of human organs and donors, stereotyping, preferential treatment of specific ethnic groups and nationalities, unethical organizational behavior, and disruptive technology and innovation that has compounded suspicions throughout the health and medical transplantation industry.

Most important were the resources I was able to gather from health and medical literature regarding organ donation and transplantation. The literature has fueled my progress in analyzing the data, allowing me to connect the various complexities, systems, disruptive behaviors, and disciplines related to the national and global crisis of organ donation and transplantation. I have used a variety of data resources from the Walden University library, which primarily include but are not limited to journal articles, magazines, newspapers, and e-books. In addition, I used online links, websites, online health and medical libraries, and YouTube.

Let us begin with this surprising but true statement by Abouna (2008).

The demand for organ transplantation has rapidly increased all over the world during the past decade

due to the increased incidence of vital organ failure, the rising success, and greater improvement in
post-transplant outcome. However, the unavailabil-
ity of adequate organs for transplantation to meet
the existing demand has resulted in major organ
shortage crises. As a result, there has been a major
increase in the number of patients on transplant
waiting lists as well as in the number of patients
dying while on the waiting list. (34)

In addition, Abouna (2008) reported a new method under
discussion.

Currently, many medical and transplant institutions
are considering alternative methods to help solve
the organ shortage, as has been achieved in the
Republic of Iran. At a recent American Congress of
Organ Transplantation (May 2007), the president
of the American Society of Transplant Surgeons,
Dr. Arthur Matas, advocated a "Regulated and
Controlled System of Living Kidney Sale." He ar-
gued that "A regulated system has the potential to
save lives and improve the quality of life. The ethical
mandate to save lives overweighs the concerns." (37)

Abouna (2008) goes on to state, "He recommended re-
evaluation of prohibition of financial incentives for both live
donors and the family of deceased donors and advocated a long-
term donor lifetime insurance coverage for any medical issue ...
In the US in 2006 there were 95,000 patients on the waiting list,
only 28,140 patients were transplanted, and 6,120 patients died
awaiting a transplant" (37).

I saw the methods and protocols as solutions to challenges
within the organ donation and transplantation crisis that have
presented new, innovative ideas I would bring to my health and
medical teams and researchers. I would then encourage those

organizations and agencies without hesitation to implement the new strategy to the way ahead. In my best judgment, a survey initiative would be the first plan of action, because statistical data that consist of national and global results would permit my research to cut right through the chase and get to the important part of the situation. Chart 5.1, Organ Crisis Solutions, is a starting point that will create more avenues to combat the current crisis.

Chart 5.1

Organ Crisis Solutions
(1) Educational programs for ICU staff and coordinators using the Donor Action System developed in several European countries, and the Donor Collaborative Action System recently developed in the US, both of which are expected to increase deceased donor (DD) organs by 20% to 30%.
(2) Appropriate use of Marginal or Extended Criteria Donors (ECD), including elderly, pediatric, diabetic, extended cold ischemia time, cardiac death, hypertension, infection with hepatitis B or hepatitis C virus, can increase the organ supply by some 20%.
(3) Acceptance of "presumed consent," a concept used in Spain and other European countries, which has increased DD organs from 14/million population per year to 34/million population per year.
(4) Use of living donors for kidney, liver, and lung transplantation. In the US, 50% of kidney transplants are from living donors (LD), with two donor deaths among 10,828 (0.03%) following laparoscopic procedure. Liver transplantation from adults to children and from adult to adult is being carried out in many transplant centers, with donor mortality of less than 1% in the US.
(5) Utilizing the concept of Paired Donation.

(6) Rewarded gifting for the family of the DD for burial expenses and for the LD for travel and lodging. It is recommended that health insurance and a tax exemption for 2 to 4 years be given to live donors for their altruistic donation.
(7) A controlled system of financial compensation be given by the government for the family of DD, as in the Kuwait System, and for live donors to an anonymous recipient, as in the Iranian System, instead of payment through greedy brokers.
(8) Encourage an "Altruistic System" of organ donation from living donors to unknown recipients, which is being developed in several countries.

Source: Abouna 2008, 37–38; Edison 2013.

I discovered another method that takes a different perspective in the arena of organ donation and transplantation processes and procedures. This involves quality-of-life (QOL) issues. I used this new method to take an in-depth look at the psychiatric challenges of reviewing organ donation recipient candidates. I would also administer this initiative in the form of a survey and include interviews to gauge the effects on donors, recipients, and family members, since the decisions made by donors aren't guaranteed, and candidates could be left dealing with the stress of disappointment.

According to Freeman III et al. (1995), "In the future, clinicians will use more sophisticated quality-of-life measures that combine subjective and objective measures in larger, widely selected samples of patients" (435). Moreover, "quality-of-life research will address the special needs of pediatric transplant recipients especially the effect of transplantation on development" (435). The importance of this method drives us toward future changes, determined by Freeman III et al.: "The future of organ transplant psychiatry depends less on immunologic and surgical advances than on 1) an increased supply of donor organs, 2) more sophisticated multicenter outcome studies, and 3) understanding of the subjective as well as objective aspects of compliance and quality of life for transplant recipients" (429). Freeman III et al. (1995) recognized, "the technical sophistication of solid organ transplantation advances, treatment regimen noncompliance has become a major cause of late post transplant mortality and morbidity," which are instruments used to determine the health and medical status of a populace. In addition, "predicting noncompliance by using psychiatric methods has gained increasing importance" (430).

In every effort to keep momentum going forward with these new organ donation solutions, the next step was to develop a survey that would allow me to effectively examine the steps leading to a psychiatric challenge of organ transplantation. The survey would address the following factors, from Freeman III et al. 1995, with answers chosen on a scale of 1 to 5, 1 being the least agreeable, and 5 being the most agreeable:

- Previous psychosocial research has attempted to be "objective" by emphasizing such factors as return to work, income, marital status, and functional disability.
- Will psychosocial factors take on greater significance in the future, especially as attention to the subjective status of patients increases?
- Many conscientious clinicians bring up an ethical dilemma, asserting that in periods of donor scarcity, even greater attention should be given to psychosocial factors, particularly the subjective aspects involved in the decision making.
- Psychiatric assessment in the future will cover as exhaustively as possible all relevant past and present clinical factors.
- Recent advances in decision theory postulate that not all factors in a major decision, such as whether to have a transplant, are of equal weight for all persons. (431–435)

Personally, I agree that "ideally future studies will integrate biomedical findings psychosocial factors and ethical analyses in the selection of candidates for organ transplantation" (Freeman III et al. 1995, 435). Thus, Freeman III et al. fathomed, "the hope for synthesis is that psychosocial research that addresses the relevant medical and ethical issues will provide the best opportunity for harmonizing the different concerns ... Optimally we can predict that surgeons and internists will see the importance of preoperative psychiatric evaluation particularly that which leads to enhanced survival rates and enhanced quality of life" (434). Still, though, "we will have data to distinguish the patient who will care for the organ optimally and have the best chance of obtaining the maximum in duration and life quality from the patient who would squander a scarce resource" (435).

On the other hand, there are activists supporting new measures that protect private transactions that pair organ donors and recipients as long as saving lives through transplantation comes first. This practice is contrary to purchasing and offering organs for sale. According to Austin (2004), "Human-transplant advocates defended the practice of some privately arranged procedures in the wake of the nation's first Internet-brokered organ transplant." She also reported, "Any sweeping prohibition on private arrangements between potential organ donors and their recipients would cost lives because the national waiting list has ballooned beyond the pool of identified donors, several organ recipients, and advocates." Consequently, Austin noted, "while opposed to the direct sale of human organs, some organ recipients said they favor financial incentives to attract more donors." The shortage of organs and donors has recipients and family members on a quest to acquire the desired needs by any means necessary.

Ethical concerns involved in this process have attracted the attention of Congress. Nevertheless, when a loved one's life is at stake and a heart, kidney, liver, lung, or other vital organ is needed to sustain life, the underlying rules and regulations of the mechanisms in place are virtually overlooked, leaving family members and recipients to chase other opportunities. "For example, Pennsylvania is piloting a $300 payment to families of deceased organ donors to help cover burial expenses ... Congress considered legislation this year that would have expanded such pilot programs." Even though, "possible test projects include allowing a recipient to donate money to charity in a donor's name—and even awarding 'medals of honor' to donors and their families" (Austin 2004, A14). Thus, for the record, "Lawmakers, however, did not pass the measure because of concern that such a system would unfairly entice low-income organ donors" (Austin 2004).

With the increasing concern regarding the short list of organ donors and the growth of the waiting list, I believe the next step to take in this matter is to create and submit a survey. Based on the survey's results, I strongly encourage conducting follow-up interviews. The logical place to start is the waiting list for organ transplants. As a variety of questions were posed to organ donors and recipients from living donor advocates, a startling surprise surfaced that shocked current views of the organ donation and transplantation processes that led to donors demonstrating unselfish devotion toward the welfare of others. This behavioral phenomenon, known as altruism, was examined by M. Austin. Austin (2004) reported that an organ donor "gave his kidney for altruistic reasons and that no money was involved." Austin also stated, "That surgery has sparked a firestorm of ethical objections from top transplant surgeons who said it undermines a time-tested system of organ allocation and opens the door for abuse." Furthermore, Austin noted we are recognizing and "allowing any kind of financial incentives would erase today's system, which guarantees pure altruism."

In this case, some believe the "argument is a bunch of hogwash, because there are always people out there who are willing to sacrifice and do it with an open heart" (Austin 2004). Nonetheless, Austin reminds us that "until cures are found for the diseases that cause organ failure, the medical community must explore other ways of getting donors to come forward," even if it resorts to unapproved methods, including ethic approval, that may be in the best interests of recipients, donors, and family members.

The examples used in this chapter pertaining to new and current methods of combating the challenges of the organ donor shortage have been very compelling. As such, the path my research has taken me thus far is the reason I elected not to address the next method last, since it might be viewed as dramatic and suspenseful—like straight out of the movies. Brace yourself, because it is absolutely chilling.

Existing circumstances have opened opportunity to a method that identifies and perpetuates the medical practices of euthanasia. Wilkinson and Savulescu (2012) stated, "the importance of this problem has led in the past to changes in attitude towards, and the legal status and clinical care of dying and dead patients, in which it contributed to the development and widespread acceptance of brain-death criteria" (32). As these changes developed, "These options range from changes to consent processes, to the use of pre-mortem extracorporeal membrane oxygenation, or organ donation euthanasia" (Wilkinson and Savulescu 2012, 33). Let's look at the emphasis behind euthanasia and determine whether it is truly a solution that meets the challenges of the human organ shortage. Table 5.1 defines the existing subject matter of euthanasia.

Table 5.1 Euthanasia Medical Description (EMD)

Medical Term	Description
Euthanasia	The intentional killing by act or omission of a dependent human being for his or her alleged benefit. (The key word here is "intentional." If death is not intended, it is not an act of euthanasia)
Voluntary Euthanasia	When the person who is killed has requested to be killed.
Non-voluntary Euthanasia	When the person who is killed made no request and gave no consent.
Involuntary Euthanasia	When the person who is killed made an expressed wish to the contrary.

Assisted Suicide	When someone provides an individual with the information, guidance, and means to take his or her own life with the intention that they will be used for this purpose. When it is a doctor, who helps another person to kill themselves it is called "physician assisted suicide."
Euthanasia by Action	Intentionally causing a person's death by performing an action, such as by giving a lethal injection.
Euthanasia by Omission	Intentionally causing death by not providing necessary and ordinary (usual and customary) care or food and water.

Source: http://www.euthanasia.com/definitions.html; Edison, 2013.

Consider this statement from the euthanasia website about what euthanasia is not.

> There is no euthanasia unless the death is intentionally caused by what was done or not done. Thus, some medical actions that are often labeled "passive euthanasia" are no form of euthanasia, since the intention to take life is lacking. These acts include not commencing treatment that would not provide a benefit to the patient, withdrawing treatment that has been shown to be ineffective, too burdensome or is unwanted, and the giving of high doses of pain-killers that may endanger life, when they have been shown to be necessary. All those are part of good medical practice, endorsed by law, when they are properly carried out. (http://www.euthanasia. com/definitions.html)

Even with extensive research, regarding Euthanasia by Action and Euthanasia by Omission, Wilkinson and Savulescu (2012) stated, "they conflict with ethical norms governing transplantation to varying degrees" (33). Furthermore, "the cost of preserving those norms will be the death or ongoing morbidity of many individuals, and this may prompt us to consider whether those principles should be revised or rejected" (33). Either way, this scenario requires additional observation and research set forth by the current health and medical guidelines. Pending the results, interviews from all parties involved might require sanctions.

Finally, with a new, innovative design, a community of African-American churches in the southeast United States set their aim on expanding organ donation through the house of God. Cleverly done, "Churches were pair-matched by average estimated income and size and then randomized to 1 of 2 interventions: one addressing organ donation between twenty-two African-American churches in Southeast Michigan" (Andrews et al. 2012, 161). It was presumed "African-Americans are disproportionately represented among those awaiting a transplant, and many are reluctant to donate their organs." The goal was "to test the effectiveness of using lay health advisors to increase organ donation among church members and see to those church members were trained to serve as lay health advisors (called peer leaders)." Andrews et al. tell us, "Peer leaders conducted organ donation discussions with church groups and showed a DVD created for this program that was tailored to African-American churches." This method "measures the primary outcome which was verified registration in the state's donor registry." In addition, it verified that "participants also completed pre/post questionnaires regarding their attitudes about organ donation."

From my observation, conducted on behalf of this research, the following results appear to demonstrate a paradigm shift. The analysis presented by Andrews et al. (2012) stated the following.

> Once clustering, baseline value, and demographics were adjusted for, the intervention and comparison groups did not differ on any of the 3 attitude scales on the posttest. In logistic regression analysis, with baseline donation status, demographics, and

church clustering controlled for, the odds of self-reported enrollment at 1-year posttest did not differ by condition (odds ratio, 1.23; 95% CI, 0.87–1.72). A total of 211 enrollments in the state registry from participating churches were verified. Of these, 163 were from intervention churches and 48 were from comparison churches. (161)

The methods used to gain the results stuck to the idea of educating African-American churches.

Motivated by the observations, the study, and the training administered by peer leaders in the African-American churches, their influence was astonishing. Above all, it carried over to the outlying communities and proved the "use of lay health advisors through black churches can increase minority enrollment in a donor registry even absent change in attitudes" (Andrews et al. 2012, 161). So far, just the surface has been scratched, because the practice was limited to African-American churches in a single community in Michigan. More so, Andrews et al. stated, "Our results also may not be generalizable to African-Americans who do not go to church or are not Christian" (166). Nevertheless, educating a community big or small is always weighed as an excellent opportunity that cannot be wasted. There is much to be gained with more communities getting on board with the objective of sharing the wealth.

CHAPTER 6
LITERATURE REVIEW

According to some health and medical officials, "Organ transplantation can treat a wide range of end-stage, life-threatening illnesses, including diseases of the heart, kidney, liver, lung, and pancreas" (Wakefield et al. 2010, 380). While the need for organs continues to increase, reports from Donate Life America (2010) indicated that "43% of Americans are undecided, reluctant, or do not wish to have their organs and tissue donated after their deaths" (as cited in Ford and Steele-Moses 2011, 405). Even more amazing, the US Department of Health and Human Services (n.d.) reported, "this problem becomes more apparent when less than 10% of all donors between January 1, 1988, and January 31, 2010, were African-American, with 25% of the U.S. African-American population comprising 29% of the organ procurement waiting list" (405). According to Wakefield et al. (2010), "individuals who held strong positive attitudes and weak negative attitudes toward organ donation were the most committed to signing a donor card" (380). Furthermore, "in order to develop more effective public health campaigns, it is critical to understand more about the attitudes and beliefs that either increase or decrease people's willingness to donate and their commitment to register their intentions" (380–381). This situation is censorious and very difficult to digest nationally and globally, since it appears to boil down to the lack of education, self-awareness, and public awareness about the need and participation in organ donation and transplantation.

Ford and Steele-Moses (2011) state it is no secret, "the issue of organ donation is relevant to nephrology nursing practice," meaning that "nurses advocate for patients' rights and are often involved in the care of patients without brain activity to sustain life (brain dead)" (405). In addition, it is important to know The Joint Commission (2007) stated, "Many regulatory agencies, including The Joint Commission and the Centers for Medicare and Medicaid Services (CMS), hold hospitals responsible for the timely referral of patients who are brain dead to organ procurement organizations to improve organ retrieval and consent rates" (as cited in Ford and Steele-Moses, 405).

Table 6.1 shows the results of a consent-rate study-specific questionnaire (SSQ).

Table 6.1 Consent Rate

Reference, date, origin	Outcome measures	Sample characteristics	Measures	Findings
Siminoff et al., 2006, USA	Willingness to donate (signed donor card)	1283 adults, mean age, 43.8 y; random sample	SSQ	Positive predictors: younger age, higher education, agrees with presumed consent, belief that hospitals need not ask family permission for organ donation; higher trust in medical system was predictive of donor status for whites, but not African-Americans.

Source: Wakefield et al. 2010, 388.

Ford and Steele-Moses (2011) articulated the value of organ donation and transplantation in health and medical innovation and technology: "The shortage of organs in America is an important health concern for nephrology nurses and the healthcare system. A profile of behaviors and beliefs that predict the willingness of African-Americans to donate organs will lend new knowledge that may help improve and increase the consent and conversion rates for organ donation among this population, and thus, add to improving the overall shortage" (409).

Wakefield et al. (2010) believe, "Future research would benefit from more sophisticated analysis of the reasons for the low numbers of organ donations worldwide." Also, a closer look at changing some of the current processes and procedures for "the older, more conventional, public health assumptions that generalized education will correct 'ignorance' and therefore 'improve behavior' may be significantly flawed" (390). Several research studies "showed that younger persons are more willing to donate their organs, and were assessments of actual donor behavior (i.e., having signed or carrying a donor card)." Wakefield et al. also "showed that persons with higher socioeconomic status and education are more willing to donate, and showed that women may be more willing to donate than are men ... researchers reported that African-American and Hispanic-American ethnicity were predictive of lower willingness to donate, and strong religious beliefs also appear to be predictive of lower willingness to donate, particularly among African-Americans" (385).

What appeared to be positive results from other cultural behaviors, based on similar processes that addressed organ donation and transplantation as a global issue, came from research "conducted in Pakistan, consisting of predominantly Muslim participants, the perception that religion allowed organ donation was a positive predictor of motivation to donate" (Wakefield et al. 2010, 385). However, "the complexity of the actual donation procedures that govern organ donation within different countries and the multiplicity of influences on these acts could not be fully captured by using the systematic review methods adopted for this" (390) research. Better yet, additional information gathered stated, "broader factors such as prevailing social and cultural norms and existing organ donation policies in different countries also significantly influence organ donation decisions" (390). Wakefield et al. believed, "continuous research and analysis, most importantly, the actions of staff of emergency departments and intensive care units, and the attitudes of family members of the deceased would also have a strong impact on organ donation rates" (390). To add to that, Wakefield et al. asserted, "It is also important for future research to begin to separate out the more modifiable individual attitudes that could reasonably be addressed by community educational intervention and those attitudes that are based in more fundamental belief systems, such as cultural and religious beliefs" (309).

Ford and Steele-Moses (2011) stated, "the voice of the living organ donor must be heard" (409) to increase "the body of knowledge on the willingness to donate by" (409) all cultures around the globe. Organ donation and transplantation in "developed countries generally meet their organ needs through cadaver organs, in developing countries like Turkey; the majority of transplantations are performed with organs taken from living relatives" (Gül et al. 2012, 1,449). Gül et al. also stated, "in developed countries 80% of donated organs are from cadavers and 20% are from living persons, yet on the other hand, in Turkey about 75%–80% are living donors" (1,449). This equates to "the number of cadaver donors for each million population is 34,6 in Spain, 21,1 in Italy, 20,9 in France, whereas in Turkey it is only 2,4" (1,449).

Gül et al. (2012) believe education, awareness, and knowledge of the organ donation and transplantation situation are contributors to a positive revelation, whereas "several factors, such as experiential, educational, social, cultural, and religious, have been affect the people's attitudes, beliefs, and behaviors toward organ donation and transplantation ... people's attitudes and beliefs toward organ donation contribute significantly to willingness to donate especially, since education provides to increase people's knowledge and awareness of this issue" (1,449).

I believe knowledge is key, and education is of paramount

importance to understanding the processes that go into decision making affecting everyone, including health and medical officials, recipients, donors, and family members. For example, cadaver donors were previously discussed as the primary means in some countries to procure organs. Long, Sque, and Addington-Hall (2008) articulated the manner of acquisition from two powerful nations: "Brain-death, whether it be brain stem death (the term used in the United Kingdom) or whole brain-death (the term used in the United States), is a prerequisite for heart-beating organ donation and is therefore a fundamental factor in the process of organ and tissue donation for transplantation" (118). Long et al. remind us that "Understanding how brain-death may be perceived by those family members approached about organ donation is an important issue to explore as biomedicine moves to expand the range of end-of-life technologies that, potentially, blur the demarcation between life and death" (119).

During this analysis, I reviewed Long et al.'s, (2008) survey to family members regarding brain-death, which stated,

> Knowledge about brain-death, by using scenarios, was carried out by Franz et al., working in the United States. Franz and colleagues carried out a cross-sectional telephone survey of 164 next-of kin of potential organ donors. They report that a sizable number (no figures provided) of donor participants were confused about whether their relative was truly dead, and furthermore, that non donating relatives had less understanding of brain-death than did donating relatives. (119)

Credit several authors who studied health and medical conditions revolving around organ donation and transplantation, concentrating on brain-death circumstances to help family members and relatives better understand how the medical diagnosis was determined. Long et al. (2008) provided the following brain-death scenarios for clarity.

> Scenario 1: A 22- or 70-year-old is in the hospital. (Two ages are listed in the scenarios. Participants were randomly sampled as to which age they would hear. This variation was done to assess whether the age of the patient indicated in the scenarios might play a part in participants' responses. It did not.) This patient is on machines (sometimes-called mechanical support or life support) that keep the heart and lungs working. The patient's brain no longer functions at all—there is no brain activity and no brain waves. (This scenario fulfills criteria for brain-death in the United States.)

> Scenario 2: A 22- or 70-year-old is in the hospital. The patient is on machines that keep the heart and lungs working. This patient's brain is so severely damaged that he/she will never recover. The patient will not wake up and will not eat or breathe on his or her own. However, there are still some brain waves left. (This scenario fulfills brain stem criteria in the United Kingdom, but would not be accepted in the United States.)

> Scenario 3: A 22- or 70-year-old is in a nursing home for 5 years after a severe brain injury. This patient is not on any life support machines and can breathe without a machine. However, the patient does need to be fed by a tube. The patient will not wake up and will never respond to people or things around him/her. There are still some brain waves left. (This patient is in a persistent vegetative state and would not be acceptable for organ donation in either the United Kingdom or the United States.) (120)

Based on these scenarios, "only 29.4% in fact correctly classified a person as dead or alive in accordance with current medical criteria and the law in the United States" (Long et al. 2008, 120). Their report concluded, "These results suggest that participants have a different concept of death than the present medical criteria, although the lack of knowledge about the medico legal definition of brain-death is clearly a factor" (121). Furthermore, "the fact that a sizable number of respondents were willing to donate the organs of people who are not legally dead is of specific importance and appears to be related to issues surrounding quality of life." Hence, who would have thought the significance of QOL had such an extraordinary role to play, with all the excitement emphasized on the lack of education provided to families and practitioners around the world. Nonetheless, "organ transplantation is one of the most efficient ways to save lives and improve the quality of life for people with end-stage organ failure" (Gül et al. 2012, 1,449).

There is still much to be gained from the vast amount of research being conducted around the world. Global health and medical experts who have conducted extensive research and analysis on organ donation and transplantation issues need to address a variety of other considerations and complex challenges. Among these challenges, health and medical officials face pathophysiological changes. Basically, pathophysiology is the study of the changes of normal mechanical, physical, and biochemical functions caused by a disease or resulting from an abnormal syndrome (http://www.en.wikipedia. org/wiki/Pathophysiology). According to Dictus et al. (2009),

> pathophysiological changes following brain-death entail a high incidence of complications including hemodynamic instability, endocrine and metabolic disturbances, and disruption of internal homeo-stasis that jeopardize potentially transplantable organs ... frequently, brain-death as a result of increased intracranial pressure after severe brain injury follows a similar pattern of rostral–caudal cerebral herniation leading to brain stem ischemia,

which mean arterial pressure rises in an effort to maintain cerebral perfusion pressure. (2)

Adverse effects from pathophysiological changes relating to brain-death have provided new insight into the study of organ donation and transplantation research. Dictus et al. (2009) affirmed, "Caring for a brain dead potential organ donor requires a shift in critical care therapy from the extensive treatment of increased intracranial pressure toward strategies to maintain donor organ function" (7). However, most importantly, I believe "a systematic and optimized critical care management increases not only the number, but also the quality of suitable organs, aiming at an optimal outcome for the recipients" (7). Important health and medical concerns revolving around pathophysiological changes illustrated in chart 6.1 and pathophysiological terms of results, shown in table 6.2, are the result of extensive research and analysis.

Chart 6.1: Pathophysiological Change and Considerations

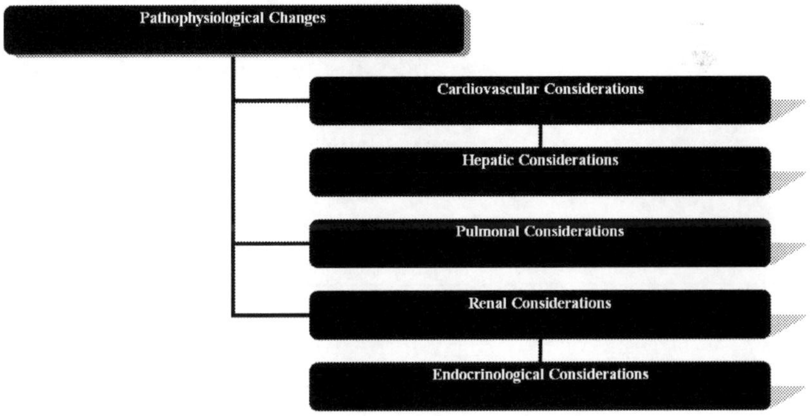

Pathophysiological Changes

Cardiovascular Considerations

Hepatic Considerations

Pulmonal Considerations

Renal Considerations

Endocrinological Considerations

Source: Dictus et al. 2009, 3–6; Edison 2013.

Table 6.2 Pathophysiological Terms and Results

Pathophysiological Term	Pathophysiological Results
Cardiovascular considerations	The hemodynamic instability is a major challenge in the treatment of brain-dead potential organ donors. Hypertension is a rare event usually occurring during the phase of cerebral herniation itself and is therefore mostly self-limitating.
Pulmonal considerations	Neurogenic pulmonary edema, pneumonia, and intense inflammatory responses make successful lung procurement in brain-dead potential organ donors challenging. However, critical care management in case of lung donation is very complex because all components of the hemodynamic model are affected.
Renal considerations	Brain-death provokes both immunological and non-immunological damage to the kidneys, which may increase the rate of delayed allograft function, the risk of acute and chronic rejection, and the incidence of renal allograft nephropathy, and may decrease recipient survival.
Hepatic considerations	The liver seems to tolerate long periods of hypo perfusion because of its large physiological reserve. Furthermore, the immunological response is weak as it is a tolerogenic organ. Nevertheless, the inflammatory processes related to brain-death and reperfusion injury to the liver lead to poor initial function of liver allografts.

| Endocrinological considerations | Dysfunction of the posterior pituitary gland with low to undetectable levels of vasopressin occurs in up to 90% of adult and pediatric organ donors and commonly results in central diabetes insipidus clinically manifested with polyuria, serum sodium concentration, urine sodium concentration, serum osmolarity, urine osmolarity, and a specific urinary weight of < 1005. Diabetes insipidus is essential to treat because it has been linked with hemodynamic instability in organ donors. |

Source: Dictus et al. 2009, 3–6; Edison 2013.

In conclusion, Long et al. (2008) stated the progress in organ donation and transplantation has taken society to new developments, whereas "Despite attempts to separate the diagnosis of brain death from the process of organ donation and transplantation, the introduction of the concept of brain death into legislation triggered a true revolution during the 1970s, which was decisive in establishing transplantation programs" (124).

Today, health and medical professions are connected globally, headed into the future bound by innovations and technologies that suggest "These findings highlight that organ donation should be included in the curriculum for all university students" (Gül et al. 2012, 1,453). In addition, Gül et al. believe that "it is necessary to review the curricula of medical and health science schools/faculties and emphasize the importance of organ donation and these subjects should be included in the all university classrooms as part of the compulsory curriculum" (1,453).

Above all, keep in mind that Long et al. (2008) confidently stated the following initiatives.

A sustained increase in the number of organs available for transplantation may never be achieved until the concepts of brain-death, brain stem death, and now non–heart-beating death (1) are debated more widely within society; (2) a greater degree of consensus is reached within health care; and (3) bereaved family members approached to donate the organs of their deceased relative have a better understanding of what these diagnoses mean. (124).

We must continue to take strides in educating the world about organ donation and transplantation, and the importance of grabbing hold of this global crisis with one unified vision committed to the human race.

CHAPTER 7

FINDINGS AND CONCLUSIONS

It surprised me to find out during my research that organ donation societies, from a global perspective, play by their own organizational rules. These rules tend to have created some cases of segregation and selective preference of who has the right to continue to live. When it comes to saving a life through an organ donor transplant program, I believe not one family in need of an organ donation would care less about the color or race of the donor. Well, let us not be too hasty, as later in this chapter, the situation climaxes to more disbelief. I believe this, because God Almighty created every human being equal. For example, most of the human organs come in pairs, yet, I do not know of any that come in threes or fours.

If a kidney is needed, there are no current criteria that ask the recipient, "Would you like your kidney from a healthy, thirty-year-old, Japanese-born, American male, or a twenty-five-year-old, healthy, African-American male." What is important is saving a life. But the double P of profit and preference has taken the lead and forced many well-deserving recipients to go to the end of the list.

Claims of a global shortage of organ donors; the lack of information and knowledge provided to family members, donors, and recipients; and the indecisiveness of family members willing to consent to donate relatives' organs remain the primary, disruptive challenges for health and medical officials. In addition, the authors articulated "findings indicated that the families faced with an organ donation request of a brain-dead loved one experienced a lasting effect long after the patient's demise regardless of their decision to donate or refusal to donate" (Manzari et al. 2012, 654). Manzari et al. stated, "These findings indicate that the essence of family experiences includes some degree of uncertainty and ambiguity, but their perception and beliefs are background dependant" (655). Although, as noted by Manzari et al. (2012), "Dissimilar to our findings, another study demonstrated that agreement or disagreement with donation had no effect on the grief process and the main variables affecting the mourning process were similar in both consenting and non-consenting families" (662).

I also found during each discussion and examination pertaining to the organ donation process, effective communication is most important when asking donor family members to consent to releasing a deceased relative's organs to save a life. Dorflinger, Auerbach, and Siminoff (2012) reported they examined "whether positive/collaborative requester behaviors elicit complementary behaviors from next of kin who were initially undecided about their willingness to donate their deceased family member's tissues." Meanwhile, further examination conducted by Dorflinger et al. provided the following analysis: "Positive requester behaviors elicited a positive response from undecided next of kin. Because many next of kin have limited knowledge about tissue donation before the request, the communication process may affect the next of kin's perceptions of donation and thus affect the likelihood of consent" (427).

Manzari et al. (2012) reported, "in line with some of these findings, researchers have asserted that a lack of understanding on brain-death contributed to conflict and dissonance." They also noted, "families who properly understood the concept of brain-death felt less conflict, guilt or uncertainty, and, dissimilar to other findings, our participants did not report increased distress over organ donation" (663).

All I have learned from the resources used to attain the data presented in my comprehensive research is acknowledged and confirmed by the following final analysis. According to Manzari et al. (2012), it is clear: "The findings of the study indicate that a request for organ donation has a significant impact on families with lasting effects after the patient's death depending on the decision made in various circumstances." They continue, "consenting and non-consenting families experience the positive effects of their decision by feelings of comfort and satisfaction alongside negative experiences such as tension, conflict, and psychological strain" (664). This is primarily why I suggest using affective communication methods to achieve positive results such as, "confirmation, approval, control, and persuasion, which led to more statements of approval by NOK" (Dorflinger et al. 2012, 435).

My research confirms "organ donation is a complex and life changing experience for families involved in any decision made" (Manzari et al. 2012, 664). They go on to state, "considering the global crisis regarding lack of donor membership, organizations have to revise their objectives by considering positive and negative family experiences in order to increase the number of consenting families." Keep in mind that "organ donation is a multifaceted issue with psychological, ethical, moral, cultural, financial, and legal components, and observing and improving every aspect could be important to the organizational success" (664).

The subject of future research dictates a requirement for "potentially informal communication skills training for tissue requesters, since future research could examine effects of such training on consent rates" (Dorflinger et al. 2012, 427). In addition, "providing an opportunity for NOK to agree more readily to donate organs in the future" (435) might establish a better relationship between requester and family member.

I have expressed unambiguously the compelling results of this extensive literature research, which "highlights the importance of family support and follow-up in an efficient healthcare system aimed at developing trust with the families and providing comfort during and after the final decision" (654). Manzari et al. find,

The organizational goal should not be focused on the safe removal of the organs and saving recipients' lives, but the human aspects of the process for both sides. Regard for the sanctity of life applies to both family groups as one gives and the other receives life. The healthcare team must promote open expression, answer questions truthfully, attempt to gain trust, maintain confidence, and help families to make the best decision. (664)

Manzari et al. (2012) eloquently and compassionately raised the level of awareness that stimulates our consciousness. At the same time, they provide a solution by unfolding the affirmed knowledge under one global umbrella that extends a universal message throughout the organ donation and transplantation health and medical industry.

CHAPTER 8

RECOMMENDATIONS

Social-impact problems involved with organ donation and transplantation have evolved into an alarming global crisis. It would be wise to begin collaborating on solutions from all levels of leadership and resources in the universal health and medical industry. Collaborators should have demonstrated ethical success rates in newfound practices aimed at gaining families' trust, in hopes the families will feel a sense of confidence and relief in their ultimate decision. I am on a quest to review all recommendations that could eventually cut in half the organ donation and transplantation shortage. My deepest emphasis will remain on educating the public about organ donor processes and procedures, and to stay focused and diligent in gaining prospective and actual donor family trust.

The importance to the difference in the two characteristics will become synchronous on successfully administering the right information about organ donation that educates the public, from future donors to actual donors. Moreover, the process is designed to further educate actual donors, which will continue to raise their levels of awareness spiritually and with integrity. I believe an actual organ donor's first point of contact is with the family, and an increase in family awareness will help to increase acquisitions and decrease the unbalanced global organ donation and transplantation waiting list.

Help has arrived from the genius of committees created by the Department of Medicine, Columbia University College of Physicians and Surgeons, New York, New York. Das and Lerner (2007) announced the following course of actions effective immediately as of 2007.

> The first three recommendations for enhancing donation are prudent and logical: (1) moving to a systems approach (i.e., disseminating best practices, improving quality assessment, and integrating end of life care to donation); (2) expanding the donor pool by moving from circulatory to neurologic criteria; and (3) improved education and decision-making opportunities. (726)

There were other considerations from the committee: "recommendations to provide potential donors with independent advocate teams and risk/benefit analyses, called for the establishment of living donor registries to provide concrete data on the short and long-term consequences of live donation" (Das and Lerner 2007, 726).

There is still room for organ donation and transplantation improvement. Researchers must leave no stone unturned to serve the best interests of donors and recipients. Das and Lerner (2007) stated, "We thus agree with the committee's recommendation opposing a pilot study of incentives because of the clearly articulated concerns over distributional inequalities, imperfect information, the commoditization of the human body, and the continuing lack of long-term information on the risks of living donation" (727).

For example, "it is hardly fair to ask an individual to donate an organ for profit when he has no access to primary care, let alone to sophisticated organ transplantation for himself" (Das and Lerner 2007, 727). More so, it is reason enough why Das and Lerner (2007) "found that the incentives were more compelling to the poorer and less educated respondents, as is asserted by the committee" (727). Yet, society tells another story, as reported by

Das and Lerner: "Citizens are expected to share sacrifice for the benefit of society both during life, for example, by registering with the Selective Service, and even after life, in the form of a sizeable, mandatory tax for those Americans with sufficiently valued estates" (728).

Das and Lerner (2007) continued, "the committee prizes the patient's right to silence to such a degree that it too quickly dismisses the counterargument: societies should be allowed to mandate some personal sacrifice if the expected outcome, such as the saving of thousands of lives, is great enough" (728).

I believe the positive takeaway, as it pertains to decision making, is that the aforementioned recommendations offer respect and dignity for our fellow human being. The fundamental concern ethically will always have to be distinguished, because organ donation and transplantation is a universal crisis. Nevertheless, Das and Lerner (2007) reminds us that "it is true that for this policy to be ethically practiced, a large and comprehensive education campaign would have to be undertaken for individuals to truly make an informed decision and to promote cultural acceptance" (728).

Other resources agree with the concerted effort to pass along valuable information to help educate donors and their families and obtain consent. Van Walraven et al. (2010) acknowledged that, "as there is a need for information before consent, we recommend donor counseling before tissue typing" (1,270) in every situation— whether it's a major organ, tissue, or bone marrow—and gaining the family's trust without compromise. It would be difficult to disagree with van Walraven et al., who stated, "Recommendations and standards should be considered for the protection of family donors" (1,272) and set in place the start of the guiding principles to winning their trust, confidence, and ultimately, their consent. Again, education, education, and more education will remain the number-one initiative that sends organizational-to-global leadership on the same path, building the universal framework to educate the world about the processes, procedures, and the blessing of life that embraces organ donation and transplantation awareness.

APPENDIX A
ACRONYMS

AD	anno Domini (the year of our Lord)
BC	before Christ
BME	black and minority ethnic
CMS	the Joint Commission and the Centers for Medicare and Medicaid Services
DD	deceased donor
ECD	marginal or extended criteria donor
EMD	euthanasia medical description
HLA	human leukocyte antigen
ICU	intensive care unit
LD	living donor
MMSL	management masters science leadership
NHBD	non-heart-beating organ donors
NNOD	National Network of Organ Donors
NOTA	National Organ Transplant Act
OPO	organ procurement organization
PAR	participatory action research
QOL	quality of life
SSQ	study-specific questionnaire
UK	United Kingdom
UNOS	United Network for Organ Sharing
USA	United States of America

APPENDIX B
ORGAN DONOR RESEARCH
PROGRAMS

Shriners Hospitals: We can rescue even more children with your donation. Please help.
http://www.shrinershospitalsforchildren.org/

Human Organs for Research: Donated organs and tissue for the advancement of medicine.
http://www.iiam.org/

Organ Donation: Share your thoughts about the responsibility of being a donor.
http://www.libertymutual.com/Responsibility/

Research Ventures: Comprehensive, customized prospect research for nonprofits.
http://www.researchventures.net/

Donor Research: Find wealthy donors with donor research solutions by WealthEngine.
http://www.WealthEngine.com

Prospect Research: International prospect research global prospect research resource
http://www.internationalprospectresearch.net/

organdonor.gov: Research reports, grants, and research.
http://www.organdonor.gov/dtcp/reports.html
http://www.organdonor.gov/dtcp/index.html

Organ Donation Research Consortium: ODRC.
http://theodrc.org/

UC Davis Health System: Department of Internal Medicine—
Transplant Research Program
http://www.ucdmc.ucdavis.edu/internalmedicine/transplant/trp.
html

Swedish Medical Center Seattle: Transplant program organ/kidney
transplant research.
http://www.swedish.org/Services/Transplant-Program/
Organ-Kidney-Transplant-Research#axzz2LNLOf8aB

Mayo Clinic Consumer Health: Unsure about donating organs for
transplant? Do not let misinformation keep you from saving lives.
http://www.mayoclinic.com/health/organ-donation/FL00077

Emory Healthcare Transplant Hospital: Transplant center program.
http://www.emoryhealthcare.org/transplant-center/index.html
(http://www.info.com/Organ%20Donor%20
Research?cb=27&cmp=316769&gclid=CIiOtP
GRw7UCFad_Qgod4QwAIw)

APPENDIX C
COMPONENTS OF GLOBAL
CHANGE SYSTEMS

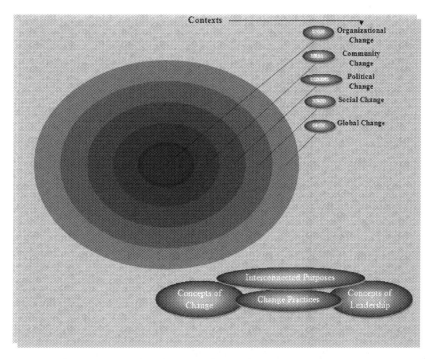

Sources: United Network for Organ Sharing (UNOS), Health Resources and Services Administration (HRSA), US Department of Health and Human Resources (USDHHS), National Network of Organ Donors (NNOD), Organ Procurement and Transplantation Network (OPTN).

APPENDIX D
GRAPHICS

Edison, J. (Designer). (2013). Organ Procurement and Transplantation Network Wait List Data [Table], created January 27, 2013, from Windows 2007 XP Professional (p.8).

Edison, J. (Designer). (2013). Public Attitudes about Financial Incentives [Table], created January 27, 2013, from Windows 2007 XP Professional (p. 17).

Edison, J. (Designer). (2013). Educational Factors of Influence and Declination [Table] created February 03, 2013, from Windows 2007 XP Professional (pp. 19-20).

Edison, J. (Designer). (2013). Organ Crisis Solution [Chart], created February 10, 2013, from Windows 2007 XP Professional (pp. 27-28).

Edison, J. (Designer). (2013). Euthanasia Medical Description [Table], created February 10, 2013, from Windows 2007 XP Professional (pp. 32-33).

Edison, J. (Designer). (2013). Pathophysiological Change and Considerations [Chart], created February 13, 2013, from Windows 2007 XP Professional (p. 43).

Edison, J. (Designer). (2013). Pathophysiological Terms and Results [Table], created February 13, 2013, from Windows 2007 XP Professional (pp. 44-45).

Edison, J. (Designer). (2013). Global Change Systems to Support Organ Donation and Transplantation [Diagram], created February 18, 2013, from Windows 2007 XP Professional (p. 59).

ANNOTATED BIBLIOGRAPHY

Abouna, G. M. "Organ Shortage Crisis: Problems and Possible Solutions." *Transplantation Proceedings* 40, no. 1 (2008): 34–38.

> This article discusses the overwhelming, peremptory, worldwide demand on organ transplantation, which has increased significantly over the last ten years. The discussion takes an in-depth look at increased improvements in post-transplant procedures. Around the globe a crisis has sparked concern because of the shortage of major organs. As a result, the recipient waiting list is growing, as is the number of recipients dying while on the organ transplantation list. A life must be lost for a life to be sustained.

Andrews, A. M., N. Zhang, J. C. Magee, R. Chapman, A. T. Langford, and K. Resnicow. "Increasing Donor Designation through Black Churches: Results of a Randomized Trial." *Progress in Transplantation* 22, no. 2 (2012): 161–167.

> This article focuses on the circumstances surrounding African-American response to get more active in representing organ donors and to support recipients awaiting a transplant. The strategy consisted of converting church members who were designated as health advisers into other leadership

positions that contributed to better educating the system. Cleverly done was installing an innovation in the African-American churches that utilized a randomized procedure to scratch the surface of African-American beliefs and commitments regarding organ donation and transplantation.

Austin, M. October 26, 2004. "Activists defend private deals to match organ donor, recipient transplant advocates say they support methods that save lives but oppose buying and selling parts: [final edition]." *Denver Post*, p. A14.

This article examines prohibition of secret arrangements among possible organ donors, recipients, and families, whereby recipients would acquire a cost. The article also addresses the large concern of the purchase and sale of major organs like hearts, kidneys, livers, and lungs for incentives like money or material possessions. The concern is even greater because of the unwanted attraction of luring the less fortunate in categories of low-income.

Baker, R. P., and V. Hargreaves. "Organ Donation and Transplantation: A Brief History of Technological and Ethical Developments." In *Bioethics—Volume 7: The Ethics of Organ Transplantation,* edited by W. Shelton and J. Balint, 1–42. Kidlington, Oxford: Elsevier Science Ltd, 2001.

The authors provide valuable information about the study, advancements, and policies surrounding bioethics and the issues that interfere with its performance. The authors believe the public principles of action will need additional transparency concerning philosophical, ideological, cultural, and sociopolitical issues. Bioethics criteria supports retaining brain-death as defining human death. With respect to human life, the simultaneous technological and ethical developments concerning organ donation and transplantation remain inconclusive.

Das, K. K., and B. H. Lerner. "Opportunities Not Taken: Successes and Shortcomings." *Kidney International* 71, no. 8 (2007): 726–729.

This article focuses on taking action on current problems in organ donation and transplantation in America that primarily concentrates on presumed consent. The article also addresses current challenges that deal with donations of many solid organs. In particular, the authors have taken the opportunity to share their perspectives and results from examining the concerns of kidney transplantation.

Dictus, C., B. Vienenkoetter, M. Esmaeilzadeh, A. Unterberg, and R. Ahmadi. "Critical Care Management of Potential Organ." *Clinical Transplantation* 23, no. 2 (2009): 2–9. http://ehis.ebscohost.com.ezp.waldenulibrary.org/ehost/detail?vid=6&sid=10bb4946-1893-4eed-9a36-1249372f637b@sessionmgr112&hid=104&bdata=JnNjb3BlPXNpdGU=.

This article discusses contingent brain-dead organ donors and change in care treatment. The growing concern about subpar care management for organ procurement has raised cause to create new strategies to meet these challenges. The authors also address concerns about pathophysiological changes stemming from brain-dead patients that enhance complications with hemodynamic instability, endocrine and metabolic disturbances, and disruption of internal homeostasis, which place transplantable organs at risk.

Doig, C. J., and G. Rocker. "Retrieving Organs from Non-Heart-Beating Organ Donors: A Review of Medical and Ethical Issues." *Canadian Journal of Anesthesia* 50, no. 10 (2003): 1069–1076.

> The article discusses ethical and medical issues surrounding the acquisition and utilization of organs from non-heart-beating organ donors (NHBD). Organizations are increasing the number of people on waiting lists for organ transplants. Support mechanisms attempt to raise the number of organs available. The non-heart-beating-organ donors program (NHBD) is a primary practice used globally in the recovery of organs. The authors discuss ethical behavior, practices, procedures, and anxiety revolving around the resolution of death and time constraints in retrieving organs capable of working successfully for transplantation. There is a shortage, and the gates are open to bidders around the world.

Dorflinger, L., S. M. Auerbach, and L. A. Siminoff. "The Interpersonal Process in Tissue Donation Requests with 'undecided' Next of Kin." *Progress in Transplantation* 22, no. 4 (2012): 427–435.

> The authors examine the interpersonal behavioral patterns of tissue requesters and the tissue donation effects on consent rates of next of kin (NOK). Whether NOK is willing to donate his or her deceased relative's tissues is the question. In addition, requester and NOK affiliation and interpersonal control are evaluated by means of communication techniques that checked NOK approval and disapproval to consenting to tissue donation.

Ford, D., and S. Steele-Moses. "Predictors for African-Americans' Willingness to Donate Organs: A Literature Review." *Nephrology Nursing Journal* 38, no. 5 (2011): 405–410.

> This article focuses on a culture labeled as disproportionate in the awareness of organ donation and transplantation procedures and requirements. The research attributes its findings to a lack of social and global education regarding the facts. The authors critically assess the prognostic behavior of African-Americans' compliance to participate in organ donation and transplantation programs with predictors such as trust, dialogue, confidence, and persuasion.

Freeman III, A. M., J. R. Westphal, L. L. Davis, and J. W. Libb. "The Future of Organ Transplant Psychiatry." *Psychosomatics* 36, no. 5 (1995): 429–437.

> The article focuses on the way ahead for organ transplant psychiatry. The research also discusses improving the election processes and procedures in obtaining candidates and anatomizing certain characteristics such as anxiety, depression, mental disturbances, and personality disorders. Additionally, merging ethical, biomedical, and psychosocial principles poses defiance toward an insufficient stock of donor organs.

Furlow, B. "Solid Organ Donation and Transplantation." *Radiologic Technology* 83, no. 4 (2012): 371–394.

> This article examines solid organ donation and transplantation and the medical imaging field. The practice includes establishing the truth through processes that diagnosis brain-dead donations. The imaging practices used assess the possible organ

donors and the waiting list recipients, rate the procured organs, and observe transplantation results. In addition, this examination covers the history of organ donations and transplantations that includes ethical practices and procedures, biological factors, and societies immensely involved in the controversial role of neurological imaging evidence that confirms clinically diagnosed brain death.

Galandiuk, S., and S. Sterioff. "The Problems of Organ Donor Shortage." *Mayo Clinic Proceedings. Mayo Clinic* 80, no. 3 (2005): 320–321.

This article describes the creation of various transplant technologies that align current stages with new steps in curtailing the organ donor and transplantation shortages for humans. The cost of the organ donor and transplantation process is very lucrative economically for chronic end-stage therapies to combat multiple organ diseases, which are of the utmost importance to health and medical providers. The current system is failing, despite tenacious attempts to stay abreast with demand. In addition, transplant medical officials have enhanced the situation by increasing restrictions in areas of age limits and related disease. Nevertheless, transplantation and organ donation have been incredibly successful.

Gül, A., H. Üstündağ, S. Purisa, and H. Gürgen. "Organ Donation: Knowledge and Attitudes of Health College and Other Departments' Students in a Turkish University." *HealthMed* 6, no. 4 (2012): 1449–1454.

This article discusses the experiences of Turkish health colleges and universities and their understanding of the organ donation processes and procedures. A questionnaire created by health and medical researchers regarding organ donation was administered to sample groups of students to determine a knowledge base. As a result, the information acquired from the survey provided percentages of how well informed students were regarding organ donation, which indicated further information and education about the subject are needed if health and medical care professionals are to advance in their progressions for the benefit of the worldwide program.

Hickman, G. *Leading Change in Multiple Contexts: Concepts and Practices in Organizational, Community, Political, Social, and Global Change Settings.* Thousand Oaks, CA: Sage Publications, Inc., 2010.

This book is an in-depth analysis of Gill Robinson Hickman's leading change in multiple contexts theory, which includes concepts and practices in organizational communities, political, social, and global change settings. Also provided is a look at how those aspects apply to the growing world of organ donor processes and procedures. The power of change is embraced by leaders in control of making organizational decisions from an ethical and moral standpoint that will affect people organization-wise, in communities, and globally. Though the book concentrates on leading change practices with different conceptual methods, leadership in the context of organ donors and transplantation has become most critical in health and medical research. Establishing global rules and regulations, educating the public, and aligning procurement are most important and the beginning to leading change.

Howard, R. J., D. L. Cornell, and L. Cochran. "History of Deceased Organ Donation, Transplantation, and Organ Procurement Organizations." *Progress in Transplantation* 22, no. 1 (2012): 6–17.

This article focuses on the history that led to the development of deceased organ donations, organ acquisition, and transplantation from an organizational viewpoint. The notion of practicing transplantation with procedures to retrieve parts from an animal or a human and using those parts in other animals or humans became a notable custom in the very distant past. Today there is a need for a constant supply of organs, and resources currently do not meet the demands. The overwhelming requirement for organs has led to the creation of specialized services and organizations, which concentrate on recognizing deceased donors, managing procurement, and contacting organ donor organizations with news and updates that availability was met for particular patients in a special category on their waiting lists.

Kierans, C., and J. Cooper. "Organ Donation, Genetics, Race and Culture: The Making of a Medical Problem." *Anthropology Today* 27, no. 6 (2011): 11–14.

This article discusses the interrelationship of organ donation and ethnicity, and the focus on the obvious unwillingness to let African-Americans and Asians in the United Kingdom become blood and organ donors. Culturally, the situation is dehumanizing, with attitudes demonstrating a lack of belief, accountability, and obligation to every human being, regardless of ethnic group. The article laid concern or blame on low supply versus high demand equals non-availability to certain groups, a preference that overrides the waiting list.

Long, T., M. Sque, and J. Addington-Hall. "What Does a Diagnosis of Brain Death Mean to Family Members Approached about Organ Donation? A Review of the Literature." *Progress in Transplantation* 18, no. 2 (2008): 118–126.

> The authors of this article examine symptoms of brain-dead donors and the complexities family members encounter pre- and post-decision–making about organ donation. The article takes an extensive look at two influential power nations' analyses of brain-death, in which one review is termed "brain-stem death" and the other which is simply brain-death. The article provides an overall picture of how biomedicine can extend the scope of end-of-life principles and applications of knowledge, which can produce an advantage to the process.

Manzari, Z. S., E. Mohammadi, A. Heydari, H. R. A. Sharbaf, M. J. M. Azizi, and E. Khaleghi. "Exploring Families' Experiences of an Organ Donation Request after Brain Death." *Nursing Ethics* 19, no. 5 (2012): 654–665.

> This article focuses on the experiences families encounter with an organ donation request after brain-death. Most of the information was collected through informal interview sessions and in-depth counseling to gauge a sense of the feelings from consenting families and those who declined organ donation. Several categories and two significant themes were covered, including serenity of eternal freedom and bitter grief, which contributed to families carrying much emotional stress long past a family member's death.

Marquardt, M. *Leading with Questions: How Leaders Find the Right Solutions by Knowing What to Ask*. 1st ed. San Francisco: Jossey-Bass, 2005.

> The author provides an extensive analysis and review of his theory regarding the study of creative leadership and the uncertain outcomes from transferring information performed by people to those in an organizational environment and if it carried over true creditable. The author proves how powerful questions asked by leaders can produce limited results with long-lasting success. Important to his set of principles is leading with questions that lead to solving problems in the complex global organization learning environment.

O'Neill, R. "Xenotransplantation: The Solution to the Shortage of Human Organs for Transplantation?" *Mortality* 11, no. 2 (2006): 211–231.

> This article examines the transplantation of animal organs and tissues into human beings with the intention of replacing human organs. The sole purpose behind this technology is based on the lingering concern of the organ supply lagging far behind global demand. In today's world, the number of human beings who die while awaiting appropriate donors continues to increase. It is no secret this shortage is the significant factor that deprives recipients of human organ transplantation. Yes, using animal organs and tissues might expand the number of available organs, but morally, we must not forget who created us and in what image.

Scheper-Hughes, N. "Keeping an Eye on the Global Traffic in Human Organs." *Lancet* 361, no 9369 (2003): 1645–1649.

This article discusses the pain, anguish, humility, and shame recipients, live donors, and families face concerning their skin colors, ethnic groups, and cultures. The contents of this article automatically categorize people in a way that places a predetermined value on their society, person, and more important, their body organs. It provides a startling analysis of information about the profit, price, and preference to organ donation and transplantation.

Shah, V., and G. Bhosale. "Organ Donor Problems and Their Management." *Indian Journal of Critical Care Medicine* 10, no. 1 (2006): 29–34.

This article focuses on the transplantation of organs from brain-deceased donors, patients standing by in intensive care units, and a discussion of cadaver programs. The article takes an in-depth look at the basic requirements for organ donation, transplantation, cost, and government facilities that aim at the number of functional organ donations and transplantation.

Shaw, R. "The Ethical Risks of Curtailing Emotion in Social Science Research: The Case of Organ Transfer." *Health Sociology Review* 20, no. 1 (2011): 58–69.

This article focuses on the organ donation and transplantation stages that concern the ethical and emotional behaviors of social researchers, donors, recipients, and their families. Overlooked are interviews and discussions surrounding anonymity procedures that dictate the affairs in relation to cooperating with the sequence of events involved with organ transfer. The article sheds light on the psychological effects of interviews, addressing experiences pre- and post-transplantation and pre- and post-counseling. A review of ethics-approval procedures for researchers intending to draw attention to vulnerable family members and recipients has led to sensitive social research interviewing and discussion that goes against the grain of positive ethical behavior by professional health and medical staffs.

Sims, S. "A Brief History of Organ Transplantation." *Penn Bioethics Journal* 6, no. 2 (2010): 10–13.

This article inspects US indoctrination into organ transplantation by taking a detailed look into the history of organ transplantation organizations. It also discusses many concerns relating to human organ transplants that have failed, transplanting animal organs in living human beings, and educating the public about organ donor processes and procedures.

Sque, M., T. Long, S. Payne, and D. Allardyce. "Why Relatives Do not Donate Organs for Transplants: 'Sacrifice' or 'Gift of Life'?" *Journal of Advanced Nursing* 61, no. 2 (2008): 134–144.

This article examines why family members decline organ donations from deceased relatives. Even if someone signs the back of his or her driver's license, indicating the desire to be an organ donor, the family can ignore that request. It could become political. A number of factors go into why family members make the decision to decline, with the primary reason being lack of education about the organ donation and transplantation processes and procedures. This article presents a detailed discussion of those issues and offers steps that lead to clarity and peace of mind.

Van Walraven, S. M., G. Nicoloso-de Faveri, U. A. I. Axdorph-Nygell, K. W. Douglas, D. A. Jones, S. J. Lee, M. Pulsipher, L. Ritchie, J. Halter, and B. E. Shaw. "Family Donor Care Management: Principles and Recommendations." *Bone Marrow Transplantation* 45, no. 8 (2010): 1269–1273.

This article explores the World Marrow Donor Association (WMDA) and its involvement in clinical transplantation and raising the comprehension of unrelated donors, particularly stem-cell donors. The authors provide in-depth analysis of WMDA standards for recruitment, counseling, workup, and subsequent donations that protect the rights of the donors.

Wakefield, C. E., K. J. Watts, J. Homewood, B. Meiser, and L. A. Siminoff. "Attitudes toward Organ Donation and Donor Behavior: A Review of the International Literature." *Progress in Transplantation* 20, no. 4 (2010): 380–391.

This article reviews the research and analysis about deceased organ donation and transplantation behaviors of individuals and their uncompromising desire to donate organs. As a result of the information gathered, people who were younger, female, and who demonstrated a higher degree of knowledge and education had positive attitudes that were overwhelmingly altruistic. In addition, they were less concerned with the devious management of the bodies of deceased donors and more inclined to participate in organ donation and transplantation programs. Nonetheless, further comprehensive research is still needed to influence a wider range of factors contributing to the much-needed positive flow of educating and learning about organ donation throughout societies worldwide.

Warren, J. "Health Horizons Medicine a Literal Gift of Life Organ Donations Are Saving Lives, but a Shrinking Donor Pool Has Caused Many to Re-Evaluate the System for Transplants." *Los Angeles Times*, October 18, 1992: 1–14.

> This article discusses the misconceptions about the shrinking donor pool, how the numbers and percentages have changed, and the desperate need for additional donors. The article also discusses waiting list concerns for specific organs and alternatives, financial incentives to donate organs, and presumed consent, which includes the automatic availability of donor organs unless instructed differently. Today it is a paradigm having more significant and demonstrable bearing than twenty years ago.

Wilkinson, D., and J. Savulescu. "Should We Allow Organ Donation Euthanasia? Alternatives for Maximizing the Number and Quality of Organs for Transplantation. *Bioethics* 26, no. 1 (2012): 32–48.

> This article connects methodologies surrounding the practices of euthanasia. The procedures that unfold the mixture of processes for organ donation euthanasia are viewed by some health and medical officials as a reasonable solution to improving the overall present practice concerning the retirement of life support on an individual. The article also steps into the realm of prolonged organ failure and death because of present organ transplantation practices.

RECOMMENDED RESOURCES

Akrivou, K., D. Bourantas, S. Mo, and E. Papalois. "The Sound of Silence—A Space for Morality? The Role of Solitude for Ethical Decision Making." *Journal of Business Ethics* 102, no. 1 (2011): 119–133.

Angeli, C., N. Valanides, and M. Papastephanou. "The Role of the Authority of the Text on Critical Thinking. *Interchange* 42, no. 3 (2011): 307–328.

Badaracco, J. L., Jr. *Defining Moments: When Managers Must Choose between Right and Right.* Boston: Harvard Business School Press, 1997.

Barker, J. A. *Paradigms: The Business of Discovering the Future.* 1st ed. New York: HarperCollins Publishers, 1992.

Barker, R. A. "The Nature of Leadership." *Human Relations* 54, no. 4 (2001): 469–494.

Bell, M. *Diversity in Organizations.* 2nd ed. Boston: South-Western Cengage Learning, 2012.

Boseman, G. "Effective Leadership in a Changing World." *Journal of Financial Service Professionals* 62, no. 3 (2008): 36–38.

Burgelman, R. A., C. M. Christensen, and S. C. Wheelwright. *Strategic Management of Technology and Innovation.* 5th ed. New York: McGraw-Hill/Irwin, 2009.

Burnes, B., and R. By. "Leadership and Change: The Case for Greater Ethical Clarity." *Journal of Business Ethics* 108, no. 2 (2012): 239–252.

Cashman, K. "Lead with Agility." *Leadership Excellence,* 28, no. 2 (2011): 6.

Chiaburu, D. S., and B. Gray. "Emotional Incompetence or Gender-Based Stereotyping?" *The Journal of Applied Behavioral Science* 44, no. 3 (2008): 293–314.

Clegg, S., M. Kornberger, and C. Rhodes. "Organizational Ethics, Decision Making, Undecidability." *Sociological Review* 55, no. 2 (2007): 393–409.

Cunliffe, A. L. "On Becoming a Critically Reflective Practitioner." *Journal of Management Education* 28, no. 4 (2004): 407–426.

Dahl, A., J. Lawrence, and J. Pierce. "Building an Innovation Community." *Research Technology Management* 54, no. 5 (2011): 19–27.

Davis, A. "Are You Talking to Your People or At Them?" *Conference Board Review* 46, no. 2 (2009): 42–46.

Di Norcia, V. "Ethics, Technology Development, and Innovation." *Business Ethics Quarterly* 4, no. 3 (1994): 235–252.

Doz, Y., J. Santos, and P. Williamson. "Diversity: The Key to Innovation Advantage. *European Business Forum* 17 (2004): 25–27.

Elder, L., and R. Paul. *The Thinkers Guide to Analytic Thinking.* Dillon Beach, CA: The Foundation for Critical Thinking, 2010.

Flood, R. L. "The Relationship of 'Systems Thinking' to Action Research." *Systemic Practice & Action Research* 23, no. 4 (2010): 269–284.

Flynn, A., and T. Mangione. "Five Steps to a Winning Project Team." *Healthcare Executive* 23, no. 1 (2008): 54–55.

Garvin, D. A. "Building a Learning Organization." *Harvard Business Review* 71, no. 4 (1993): 78–91.

Gayle, D. "An Organ Is Sold Every Hour, WHO Warns: Brutal Black Market on the Rise again Thanks to Diseases of Affluence." *Mail Online* (May 27, 2010).

Gilbert, C., M. Eyring, and R. N. Foster. "Two Routes to Resilience." *Harvard Business Review* 90, no. 12 (2012): 65–73.

Godfrey, P. "Using Systems Thinking to Learn to Deliver Sustainable Built Environments." *Civil Engineering & Environmental Systems* 27, no. 3 (2010): 219–230.

Goldsmith, M., and J. Balash. "High-Value Strategies." *Leadership Excellence* 26, no. 6 (2009): 12–13.

Goleman, D., and R. Boyatzis. "Social Intelligence and the Biology of Leadership." *Harvard Business Review* 86, no. 9 (2008): 74–81.

Harkins, P. "High-Impact Team Leaders." *Leadership Excellence* 25, no. 12 (2006): 3–4.

Hoy, H., S. Alexander, and K. H. Frith. "Effect of Transplant Education on Nurses' Attitudes toward Organ Donation and Plans to Work with Transplant Patients." *Progress in Transplantation* 21, no. 4 (2011): 317–321.

Joiner, B. "Guide to Agile Leadership." *Industrial Management* 51, no. 2 (2009): 10–15.

Jones-Burbridge, J. A. "Servant Leadership." *Corrections Today* 73, no. 6 (2012): 45–47.

Joseph, E. E., and B. E. Winston. "A Correlation of Servant Leadership, Leader Trust, and Organizational Trust." *Leadership & Organization Development Journal* 26, no. 1/2 (2005): 6–22.

Jung, H., I. Egyed-Zsigmond, L. Hecser, and K. Brînzaniuc. "Attitudes and Preferred Information Sources in Medical Students and Family Doctors Regarding Organ Donation and Transplantation." *Acta Medica Marisiensis* 57, no. 6 (2011): 649–652.

Kiechel III, W., and M. Rosenthal. "The Leader as Servant. *Fortune* 125, no. 9 (1992): 121-122.

Küpers, W. "Learning Organization." In *Encyclopedia of Leadership*, 2004:882-888

Levitt, T. "Global Competition Spells the End of Domestic Territoriality, No Matter How Diminutive the Territory May Be." *McKinsey Quarterly*, no. 3 (1984): 2–20.

Lubin, D. A., and D. C. Esty. "The Sustainability Imperative." *Harvard Business Review* 88, no. 5 (2010): 42–50.

Masood, S. A., S. S. Dani, N. D. Burns, and C. J. Backhouse. "Transformational Leadership and Organizational Culture: The Situational Strength Perspective." *Proceedings of the Institution of Mechanical Engineers* 220, no. B6 (2006): 941–949.

McLaurin, J. R., M. B. Al Amri. "Developing an Understanding of Charismatic and Transformational Leadership." *Proceeding of the Academy of Organizational Culture, Communications, and Conflict* 13, no. 2 (2008): 15–19.

McWhinney, W. "Alternative Realities: Their Impact on Change and Leadership." *Journal of Humanistic Psychology* 24, no. 4 (1984): 7–38.

Meadows, D. H. *Thinking in Systems.* White River Junction, VT: Chelsea Green Publishing Company, 2008.

Mella, P. "Systems Thinking: The Art of Understanding the Dynamics of Systems." *International Journal of Learning* 15, no. 10 (2009): 79-88.

Mendenhall, M. E., J. S. Osland, A. Bird, G. R. Oddou, and M. L. Mazvenski. *Global Leadership: Research, Practice and Development.* New York and Abingdon, Oxon: Routledge, 2008.

Molinsky, A. "Cross-Cultural Code-Switching: The Psychological Challenges of Adapting Behavior in Foreign Cultural Interactions." *Academy of Management Review* 32, no. 2 (2007): 622–640.

Moorlock, G., H. Draper, and S. R. Bramhall. "Liver Transplantation Using 'Donation after Circulatory Death' Donors: The Ethics of Managing the End-of-Life Care of Potential Donors to Achieve Organs Suitable for Transplantation." *Clinical Ethics* 6, no. 3 (2011): 134–139.

Nidumolu, R., C. K. Prahalad, and M. R. Rangaswami. "Why Sustainability Is Now the Key Driver of Innovation." *Harvard Business Review* 87, no. 9 (2009): 56–64.

Northouse, P. G. *Leadership: Theory and Practice.* 5th ed. Thousand Oaks, CA: Sage Publication, Inc., 2010.

Obama, B. "Yes, Our Path Is Harder—but It Leads to a Better Place." *Vital Speeches of the Day* 78, no. 10 (2012): 341–345.

Padela, A. I., S. Rasheed, G. J. W. Warren, H. Choi, and A. K. Mathur. "Factors Associated with Positive Attitudes toward Organ Donation in Arab Americans." *Clinical Transplantation* 25, no. 5 (2011): 800–808.

Reynolds, S. J. "Perceptions of Organizational Ethicality: Do Inflated Perceptions of Self Lead to Inflated Perceptions of the Organization?" *Journal of Business Ethics* 42, no. 3 (2003): 253–266.

Robinson, A. G., and D. M. Schroeder. "Big Results from Small Ideas. *Industrial Management* 47, no. 3 (2005): 21–26.

Rodríguez-Arias, D., M. J. Smith, and N. M. Lazar. "Donation after Circulatory Death: Burying the Dead Donor Rule." *The American Journal of Bioethics: AJOB* 11, no. 8 (2011): 36–43.

Ryan, J. *Learning Agility Equals Leadership Success,* 2009.

Sabir, M. S., J. J. Iqbal, K. U. Rehman, K. A. Shah, and M. Yameen. "Impact of Corporate Ethical Values on Ethical Leadership and Employee Performance." *International Journal of Business & Social Science* 3, no. 2 (2012): 163–171.

Salim, A., C. Berry, E. J. Ley, D. Schulman, S. Navarro, S., and L. S. Chan. "Utilizing the Media to Help Increase Organ Donation in the Hispanic American Population." *Clinical Transplantation* 25, no. 6 (2011): 622–628.

Schein, E. H. *The Corporate Culture Survival Guide.* San Francisco: Jossey-Bass, 1999.

Senge, P. M. *The Fifth Discipline: The Art & Practice of the Learning Organization.* 2nd ed. New York: Currency Doubleday, 2006.

Shipton, H., D. Fay, M. West, M. Patterson, and K. Birdi. "Managing People to Promote Innovation." *Creativity & Innovation Management* 14, no. 2 (2005): 118–128.

Sull, D., and K. M. Eisenhardt. "Simple Rules for a Complex World." *Harvard Business Review* 90, no. 9 (2012): 68–74.

Taylor, B. B. "True Purpose." *Christian Century* 118, no. 6 (2001): 30.

Tichy, N., and W. Bennis. "Making Judgment Calls." *Harvard Business Review* 85, no. 10 (2007): 94–102.

Trompeta, J. A., B. A. Cooper, N. L. Ascher, S. M. Kools, C. M. Kennedy, and J. L. Chen. "Asian American Adolescents' Willingness to Donate Organs and Engage in Family Discussion about Organ Donation and Transplantation." *Progress in Transplantation* 22, no. 1 (2012): 33–41.

Utterback, J. M., and H. J. Acee. "Disruptive Technologies: An Expanded View." *International Journal of Innovation Management* 9, no. 1 (2005): 1–17.

Vargas-Hernández, J. G., M. R. Noruzi, and S. Narges. "Risk or Innovation, Which One Is Far More Preferable in Innovation Projects?" *International Journal of Marketing Studies* 2, no. 1 (2010): 233–244.

Wagner, T. R., and C. Manolis. "The Fear Associated with Blood and Organ Donation: An Explication of Fright and Anxiety." *Progress in Transplantation* 22, no. 2 (2012): 200–206.

Wolfe, R. A., E. C. Roys, and R. M. Merion. "Trends in Organ Donation and Transplantation in the United States, 1999–2008." *American Journal of Transplantation* 10, no. 4 (2010): 961–972.

Wong, L. P. "Knowledge, Attitudes, Practices, and Behaviors Regarding Deceased Organ Donation and Transplantation in Malaysia's Multi-Ethnic Society: A Baseline Study." *Clinical Transplantation* 25, no. 1 (2011): 22–31.

Internet Sources

Farlex. "Human Leukocyte Antigen (HLA)." *The Free Dictionary,* January 1, 2013. http://medical-dictionary.thefreedictionary.com/human leukocyte antigen (accessed February 10, 2013).

Health Resources and Services Administration. "Data." Organ Procurement and Transplantation Network. http://optn.transplant.hrsa.gov/data (accessed February 10, 2013).

Schindler, Bobby. "Euthanasia Suicide Mercy-Killing Right-to-Die Physician Assisted Suicide Living Wills Research." *Euthanasia.com,* August 31, 2011. http://euthanasia.com/ (accessed February 18, 2013).

Schooley Mitchell. http://www.schooleymitchell.com/english/charity/och_history.php (accessed February 3, 2013).

The Journal of the American Medical Association (JAMA). "Consensus Statement on the Live Organ Donor," January

1, 2013. http://jama.jamanetwork.com/article.aspx?articleid=193360 (accessed February 3, 2015).

Varmus, Harold. "Comprehensive Cancer Information." *National Cancer Institute.* http://www.cancer.gov/ (accessed February 10, 2013).

WordPress and Stargazer. *Thenationalnetworkoforgandonors.org.* January 1, 2013. http://www.thenationalnetworkoforgandonors.org/about.html (accessed February 10, 2013).

Printed in the United States
By Bookmasters